Contemporary Diagnosis and Management of

Neonatal Respiratory Diseases®

Second Edition

Thomas N. Hansen, MD

Chairman, Department of Pediatrics,
The Ohio State University, and
Medical Director, Children's Hospital, Columbus, Ohio

Timothy R. Cooper, MD

Assistant Professor of Pediatrics and Ethics,
Department of Pediatrics and Center for Medical Ethics
and Health Policy,
Baylor College of Medicine, Houston, Texas

Leonard E. Weisman, MD

Professor of Pediatrics, Baylor College of Medicine;
Head, Section of Neonatology, Baylor College of Medicine;
Chief, Neonatology Service, Texas Children's Hospital;
and Director, Neonatal-Perinatal Medicine Fellowship,
Houston, Texas

Published by Handbooks in Health Care Co., Newtown, Pennsylvania, USA

This book has been prepared and is presented as a service to the medical community. The information provided reflects the knowledge, experience, and personal opinions of all the contributing authors, but especially of the three co-editors, Thomas N. Hansen, MD, Timothy R. Cooper, MD, and Leonard E. Weisman, MD.

This book is not intended to replace or to be used as a substitute for the complete prescribing information prepared by each manufacturer for each drug. Because of possible variations in drug indications, in dosage information, in newly described toxicities, in drug/drug interactions, and in other items of importance, reference to such complete prescribing information is definitely recommended before any of the drugs discussed are used or prescribed.

International Standard Book Number: 1-884065-23-6

Library of Congress Catalog Card Number: 97-75089

Table of Contents

Chapter 5: Subacute and Chronic Acquired Parenchymal Lung Diseases

Chapter 6: Congenital Diseases Affecting the Lung Parenchyma

Chapter 7: Diseases Affecting the Diaphragm and Chest Wall

Chapter 8: Diseases of the Upper Airway

Chapter 9: Control of Breathing in the Neonate

Chapter 10: Respiratory Therapy–General Considerations

Chapter 11: Nutritional and Gastrointestinal Support for the Infant with Respiratory Distress

Chapter 12: Ethical Considerations

Chapter 13: Discharge Planning

Contributors

Steven A. Abrams, MD
Associate Professor of Pediatrics, Baylor College of Medicine,
Houston, Texas

James M. Adams, Jr, MD
Associate Professor of Pediatrics, Baylor College of Medicine;
Medical Director, Special Care Nurseries,
Texas Children's Hospital, Houston

Carol L. Berseth, MD
Associate Professor of Pediatrics and Gastroenterology,
Baylor College of Medicine

Gerardo Cabrera-Meza, MD
Assistant Professor of Pediatrics, Baylor College of Medicine

Timothy R. Cooper, MD
Assistant Professor of Pediatrics and Ethics, Department of Pediatrics
and Center for Medical Ethics and Health Policy, Baylor College of Medicine

Stephen J. Elliott, MD
Associate Professor of Pediatrics and Physiology,
Principal Investigator, Cardiovascular Research Center,
Medical College of Wisconsin, Milwaukee, Wisconsin

Joseph A. Garcia-Prats, MD
Associate Professor of Pediatrics and Ethics, Department of Pediatrics
and Center for Medical Ethics and Health Policy, Baylor College of Medicine;
Co-Director, Perinatal Outreach Program,
Texas Children's Hospital, Houston, Texas

Alfred L. Gest, MD
Assistant Professor of Pediatrics, Baylor College of Medicine

Michael R. Gomez, MD
Neonatologist, Victoria, Texas

Charleta Guillory, MD
Assistant Professor of Pediatrics, Baylor College of Medicine

Thomas N. Hansen, MD
Chairman, Department of Pediatrics, The Ohio State University;
Medical Director, Children's Hospital, Columbus, Ohio

Michelle M. Heng, MD
Pediatrician, Houston, Texas

William Scott Jarriel, MD
Neonatologist, Houston, Texas

Karen E. Johnson, MD
Assistant Professor of Pediatrics, Baylor College of Medicine

Joyce M. Koenig, MD
Assistant Professor of Pediatrics, Baylor College of Medicine

Steven R. Leuthner, MD
Assistant Professor of Pediatrics, Medical College of Wisconsin
Milwaukee, Wisconsin

Alicia A. Moïse, MD
Assistant Professor of Pediatrics, Baylor College of Medicine

Richard J. Schanler, MD
Professor of Pediatrics, Director, Neonatal Nutrition Service,
Baylor College of Medicine

Virginia F. Schneider, PA-C
Instructor in Pediatrics and Family and Community Medicine,
Clinical Coordinator, Physician Assistant Program,
Baylor College of Medicine

Michael E. Speer, MD
Associate Professor of Pediatrics, Baylor College of Medicine;
Director of Nurseries, The Methodist Hospital;
Director of Nurseries, St. Luke's Episcopal Hospital, Houston, Texas

Kerry D. Stewart, MD
Neonatologist, Hattiesburg, Mississippi

Christina J. Valentine, RD
Medical Student, Baylor College of Medicine

Mary E. Wearden, MD
Assistant Professor of Pediatrics, Baylor College of Medicine

Leonard E. Weisman, MD
Professor of Pediatrics, and Head, Section of Neonatology,
Baylor College of Medicine;
Chief, Neonatology Service, Texas Children's Hospital;
Director, Neonatal-Perinatal Medicine Fellowship, Houston, Texas

Stephen E. Welty, MD
Assistant Professor of Pediatrics, Baylor College of Medicine

Foreword

In recent years, we have witnessed an explosion of new information about the pathophysiologic processes involved in diseases of the respiratory system of the newborn. This has led to improved treatments, such as surfactant replacement, that have markedly reduced morbidity and mortality in this vulnerable population.

In this second edition of this book, we review the epidemiology, pathophysiology, presentation, management, and outcomes for respiratory disorders affecting the newborn. In addition, we have provided updated reviews of pulmonary physiology and ventilatory and nonventilatory management of respiratory distress. Finally, we have stressed supportive care that is necessary to optimize outcome by including sections on nutritional and gastrointestinal support, communications with parents, ethical considerations, and discharge planning.

To a large extent, this book represents a compilation of lectures and handouts provided to postdoctoral fellows, pediatric residents, medical students, and nurses working in the nurseries of the Baylor College of Medicine Affiliated Hospitals. A list of suggested readings accompanies each chapter. Although comprehensive, this book is not meant to be an exhaustive review of the literature on any topic. It simply represents a starting point, and the reader should obtain additional information where appropriate.

The authors of this text were all students of Dr. Arnold J. Rudolph, the consummate teacher of neonatology. They wish to acknowledge his immeasurable contributions to their education, lives, and careers.

Thomas N. Hansen, MD
Timothy R. Cooper, MD
Leonard E. Weisman, MD

Chapter 1

Anatomy and Development of the Lung

Neonatal lungs are not simply small versions of the adult organ. Especially in the case of the preterm infant, respiratory disease occurs in a setting of incomplete development of the tracheobronchial system or the pulmonary vasculature. Much of the respiratory physiology observed at the bedside of the sick neonate can be accounted for by underdeveloped or maldeveloped alveolar and vascular architecture.

Alveolar Development

The tracheobronchial airway system begins as an embryonic lung bud, which then continuously divides and branches, steadily penetrating the mesenchyma and progressing toward the periphery. The process is described in five phases (Figure 1).

Embryonic Phase (Through Week 5)

Development of proximal airways. The lung bud arises from the foregut 23 to 26 days after fertilization. Abnormal lung bud development at this very early stage can result in tracheal agenesis/stenosis or in tracheoesophageal fistula. Pulmonary sequestrations develop from accessory lung buds. If an accessory lung bud develops early, the sequestration and normal lung will share a common pleura. As many as 30% of infants with congenital diaphragmatic hernia (CDH) will have pulmonary sequestrations.

Pseudoglandular Phase (Weeks 5 Through 16)

Development of lower conducting airways. In this phase, 20 generations of conducting airways form. The first eight

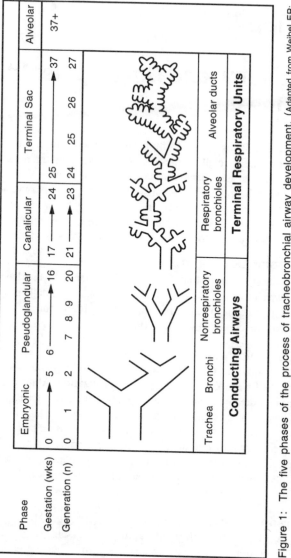

Phase	Embryonic	Pseudoglandular		Canalicular	Terminal Sac		Alveolar
Gestation (wks)	0 ▲ 5	6 ▲ 16		17 ▲ 24 25 ▲ 37			37+
Generation (n)	0 1 2	7 8 9 20		21 ▲ 23 24 25	26 27		
	Trachea Bronchi	Nonrespiratory bronchioles		Respiratory bronchioles	Alveolar ducts		
		Conducting Airways			**Terminal Respiratory Units**		

Figure 1: The five phases of the process of tracheobronchial airway development. (Adapted from Weibel ER: *Morphometry of the Human Lung.* Berlin, Springer-Verlag, 1963, p 111.)

generations (the bronchi) ultimately acquire cartilaginous walls. Generations 8 to 20 comprise the nonrespiratory bronchioles, which do not possess cartilage. By the end of this phase, development of preacinar structures (which form the conducting airways) is largely complete. All the time, airways are accompanied by surrounding lymph vessels and bronchial capillaries. The origin of bronchogenic cysts detected in infancy can be traced to the formation of bronchi with dysgenic cartilage. A more common disorder, congenital lobar emphysema, may have a similar origin but is clinically characterized by partial airway closure and gas trapping in downstream alveoli.

Closure of the diaphragm also occurs during the pseudoglandular phase. If closure is delayed past 8 to 10 weeks' gestation, migration of bowel into the thoracic cavity is possible, resulting in CDH. The pathophysiology of CDH involves more than a space-occupying lesion with compression of developing lung. Associated pulmonary hypoplasia is characterized by decreased numbers of tracheobronchial generations and alveoli. A decreased number of pulmonary arteries, plus abnormal extension of muscle into acinar arterioles, account for the persistent pulmonary hypertension that often occurs with CDH. The earlier in gestation that bowel migrates into the chest, the more severe the lung hypoplasia.

Canalicular Phase (Weeks 17 Through 24)

Formation of gas-exchanging acini. Continued branching of the airways forms respiratory bronchioles that represent the first gas-exchanging sites (acini) within the tracheobronchial tree (generations 21 to 23). During this phase, the relative amount of connective tissue diminishes. Development of pulmonary capillaries precedes acinar development, and by the end of the canalicular phase, the capillaries have begun to appose the acini. Lung function of infants born around 24 weeks greatly depends on the degree to which acinar development and acinus-capillary coupling have occurred.

Terminal Sac Phase (Weeks 24 Through 37)

Development of acini. The rudimentary primary saccules divide into subsaccules and alveoli, while the interstitium continues to dissipate. Capillary invasion becomes more extensive and leads to an exponential increase in alveolar-blood barrier surface area. Positive pressure ventilation of infants born early in the terminal sac phase can result in pulmonary interstitial emphysema, a condition in which microscopic rupture of acini leads to accumulation of small bubbles of air within the relatively thick interstitium. Incomplete invasion of the acini by surrounding capillaries provides an anatomic basis for the ventilation-perfusion mismatching that contributes to hyaline membrane disease and other parenchymal diseases.

Alveolar Phase (Week 37 to Age 3 Years)

Continued alveolar proliferation and development. In the final phase, which begins between 30 and 37 weeks, subsaccules become alveoli as a result of thinning of acinar walls, dissipation of interstitium, and invagination of alveoli by pulmonary capillaries. Ultimately, alveoli attain a polyhedral shape.

Vascular Development

The lung is supplied by the systemic bronchial circulation and the pulmonary circulation. Systemic bronchial arteries supply the conducting airways, visceral pleura, connective tissue, pulmonary arteries, and pulmonary sequestration tissue. By contrast, the pulmonary circulation participates in gas exchange and supplies arterial blood to cystic adenomatoid malformations.

Beyond 16 weeks' gestation, preacinar pulmonary arteries increase only in length and diameter, whereas intra-acinar arteries proliferate. Muscularization of fetal pulmonary arteries is confusing but important to the understanding of persistent pulmonary hypertension, a condition caused by failure of the pulmonary vasculature to relax normally in the postdelivery period. Simply put, arteries <100 μm in diameter are nonmuscular, arteries 100 to 180 μm are transitional, and those >180 μm are muscular. For any given size muscular artery, wall thickness *as a fraction of total vessel diameter* is greater in the fetus than in the adult. Wall thickness as a fraction of total diameter remains constant through the second half of gestation, so as the number of vessels increases, the total amount of pulmonary vascular smooth muscle increases. This explains, in part, why persistent pulmonary hypertension is largely a phenomenon of term and near-term infants.

During the second half of gestation, the number of arteries increases tenfold, but blood flow increases by only two- to threefold and reaches only 7% of combined ventricular output near term. The increase in smooth muscle content and hypoxic vasoconstriction together act to limit pulmonary blood flow until after delivery. At birth, oxygenation, mechanical distention of the lung, and endothelial-dependent mechanisms all contribute to a dramatic decrease in pulmonary vascular resistance and increased pulmonary blood flow.

Conclusion

The degree of vascular and alveolar development within the lung modifies the disease process in most neonatal respiratory disorders. In some circumstances, such as CDH, aberrant development is itself the primary cause of abnormal lung function.
By Stephen J. Elliott, MD, and Steven R. Leuthner, MD

Suggested Reading

Hansen TN, Corbet AJ: Lung development and function. In: Taeusch HW, Ballard RA, Avery ME, eds. *Schaffer and Avery's Diseases of the Newborn.* 6th ed. Philadelphia, WB Saunders Co, 1991.

Hislop A, Reid L: Growth and development of the respiratory system. In: Davis JA, Dopping J, eds. *Scientific Foundations of Paediatrics.* London, Heineman, 1974.

Hislop A, Reid L: Development of the acinus in the human lung. *Thorax* 1974;29:90.

Langston C, Kida K, Reed M, et al: Human lung growth in late gestation and in the neonate. *Am Rev Respir Dis* 1984;129:607-613.

Murray JF: In: *The Normal Lung.* Murray JF, ed. Philadelphia, WB Saunders Co, 1986.

Chapter 2

Respiratory Physiology

Lung Mechanics

Breathing, the physical act of moving gas in and out of the lung, is affected by mechanical properties of the tissues of the lung, the chest wall, and the inspired gas (Table 1).

Elastic Forces

The lung is composed of elastic tissues that resist stretching. Consequently, the distending pressure needed to inflate the lung increases with the volume of inflation (Figure 1). The chest wall, like the lung, contains elastic tissues and also has a compliance, C_{cw}. The lung and chest wall together determine the elastic properties of the entire respiratory system (Figure 2).

The *lung* has no innate resting volume, and if isolated from the *chest wall*, it collapses completely. As distending pressure increases from zero, lung volume increases proportionally. The chest wall has a resting volume (volume at distending pressure equal to zero) that is greater than zero. This volume is determined by the fixed volume of the rib cage. Lowering the volume of the chest cage below its resting value requires a negative distending pressure to overcome this elastic recoil. Increasing the volume of the chest cage above this resting volume requires a positive distending pressure.

Together, the lung and chest wall make up the *respiratory system*. At rest, the tendency for the chest wall to

Table 1: Pulmonary Function in Term Newborns

Lung Volumes	Measurement
Functional residual capacity	30 mL/kg
Tidal volume	6 mL/kg
Dead space volume	2 mL/kg
Ventilatory Measurements	**Measurement**
Respiratory rate	35 breaths/min
Minute ventilation	210 mL/kg/min
Alveolar ventilation	140 mL/kg/min
Mechanics	**Measurement**
Respiratory system compliance	3 mL/cm H_2O
Lung compliance	4 mL/cm H_2O
Chest wall compliance	20 mL/cm H_2O
Total inspiratory resistance	0.069 cm H_2O/mL/s
Total expiratory resistance	0.097 cm H_2O/mL/s
Inspiratory time constant	0.2 s
Expiratory time constant	0.3 s

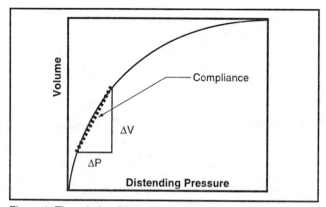

Figure 1: The relationship between distending pressure and volume of inflation for the lung is nearly linear over the volume range encompassed by normal breathing. At higher volumes of inflation, the curve becomes flatter as the lung reaches its elastic limit. The slope of the pressure-volume curve for the lung, $\Delta V/\Delta P$, is a measure of lung distensibility or compliance (C_L). Accordingly, the pressure (P) required to overcome lung elastic forces at any lung volume (V) is inversely related to compliance, $P = V/C_L$. A poorly compliant lung requires a large increase in pressure to produce a given change in volume.

Figure 2: The lung and chest wall are coupled at their pleural surfaces and together form the respiratory system. The pressure inside the lung is alveolar pressure (Palv) while the pressure surrounding the lung is pleural pressure (Ppl). Therefore, the distending pressure for the lung is Palv - Ppl. Similarly, the pressure 'inside' the chest wall is pleural pressure, the surrounding pressure is atmospheric pressure (Patm), and the distending pressure is Ppl - Patm. The distending pressure for the respiratory system is the sum of the distending pressures for the lung and chest wall or Palv - Patm.

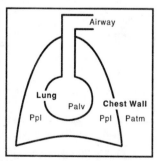

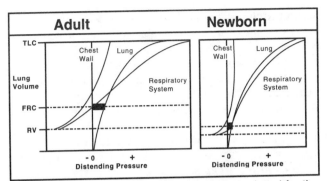

Figure 3: Idealized pressure-volume curves are plotted for the lung and chest wall separately and then for the complete respiratory system (lung + chest wall). Lung volume is normalized to total lung capacity (TLC). Other volumes shown are functional residual capacity (FRC) and residual volume (RV). The distending pressures for the lung, chest wall, and respiratory system are listed in Figure 2. (Adapted from Hansen TN, Corbet AJ. In: Taeusch HW, et al, eds. *Schaffer and Avery's Diseases of the Newborn*. 5th ed. Philadelphia, WB Saunders, 1991.)

expand is balanced by the tendency for the lung to collapse. The point at which these two forces are exactly equal and opposite is the resting lung volume or functional residual capacity (FRC). At this point, the distending pressure across the respiratory system is zero (Figure 3). Exhalation below FRC requires a negative distending pressure (active expiration). The bony structures of the chest wall limit exhalation to a minimum volume—residual volume (RV). Inflation of the thorax above FRC initially requires that work be done only to overcome the elastic forces of the lung. However, as inflation continues beyond the resting volume for the chest wall, the distending pressure must overcome the elastic recoil of both the lung and chest wall. When corrected for size of the lung, the compliance of the lung of the newborn is similar to that of the adult, but the chest wall compliance is greater. Consequently, the infant has a lower FRC and RV.

Resistance

Resistance to breathing results from friction generated by movement of gas (airway resistance) and movement of tissues (viscous tissue resistance).

Airway resistance. Friction develops as molecules of gas slide over one another and past airway walls. Gas flow through a tube requires a pressure gradient to overcome these friction forces. The magnitude of the pressure gradient is proportional to the rate of flow times a constant termed 'resistance.' Gas flow through a tube may be *laminar* or *turbulent* (Figure 4).

Turbulent flow typically occurs at high rates of gas flow or at points where airways change size or branch. In the lung, the highest rate of gas flow is in the trachea, since all of the gas entering and leaving the lung must pass through the trachea. Conversely, the lowest rates of flow will occur in small peripheral airways, since each small airway is exposed to only a fraction of the total gas flow. Therefore, flow in small airways tends to be laminar, and turbulent flow tends to occur in large central airways.

Both types of flow can occur in the lung at the same time, so the total pressure gradient required to sustain flow can be summarized by:

$$\Delta P = K_1 \times \dot{V} + K_2 \times \dot{V}^2$$

Differences between laminar and turbulent flow can be used to ascertain the site of airway obstruction. K_1 is directly related to viscosity of the gas, while K_2 is related to the density of the gas (Figure 4). Therefore, in a patient with large airway obstruction, such as croup or tracheal stenosis, decreasing the density of the inspired gas by changing from a mixture of oxygen in nitrogen to a mixture of oxygen in helium, Heli-Ox, should lower resistance to breathing and improve gas flow. Conversely,

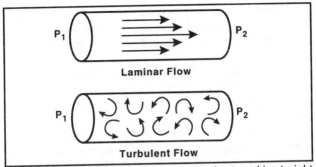

Figure 4: During laminar flow, gas molecules travel in straight lines, with the faster-moving molecules near the center of the gas stream. For laminar flow, the pressure gradient, $\Delta P = P_1 - P_2$, is directly proportional to the rate of flow ($\dot{V}$): $\Delta P = K_1 \times \dot{V}$. K_1, the resistance term, increases with length of the airway and viscosity of the gas and decreases with the fourth power of the radius of the airway. During turbulent flow, gas molecules move chaotically and the velocity of flow is the same across the stream. ΔP is proportional to the flow rate squared: $\Delta P = K_2 \times \dot{V}^2$. K_2, the resistance term, is more complicated and increases with length of the airway and density of the gas and decreases with the fifth power of the radius of the airway. (Adapted from Comroe JH, et al. *The Lung.* 2nd ed. Chicago, Year Book Medical Publishers, 1962.)

if the obstruction is in small airways, then changing gas density will not affect airway resistance and work of breathing.

Airway resistance is directly related to the length of the airway but is related to the fourth power of the airway radius. Therefore, during inspiration, as airways both dilate and lengthen, the dominant effect is to lower airway resistance. Similarly, during expiration, airways are compressed and resistance increases. Consequently, *expiratory airway resistance is greater than inspiratory airway resistance*.

Viscous tissue resistance. Viscous tissue resistance develops because of friction between tissues in the lung and chest wall. It accounts for roughly 20% of resistive forces in the newborn.

Total resistance. The total respiratory resistance is the sum of airway resistance and tissue resistance. Approximately 80% of total resistance results from airway resistance, and in the newborn about 50% of that is nasal resistance.

In practice, gas flow in the lung is assumed to be laminar, and tissue and airway resistances are lumped as the total resistance of the respiratory system (R). The pressure required to overcome resistive forces is expressed as the product of gas flow rate, $\dot{V}$, times resistance, R: $P = \dot{V} \times R$.

Inertance. During breathing, work must also be performed to accelerate gas and tissues. Generally, inertance losses are negligible compared with resistance losses and are ignored.

Dynamic Interaction

The *total driving pressure* required to move gas in or out of the lung is determined by the sum of the pressures needed to overcome elastic, resistive, and inertial forces of the lung and chest wall.

Spontaneous breathing. For spontaneous breathing, the driving pressure is simply alveolar pressure minus pleural pressure (the distending pressure across the lung [Figure 2]). During a spontaneous inspiration, inspiratory muscles of the chest wall and the diaphragm contract, increasing thoracic volume and decreasing intrapleural pressure. Decreased intrapleural pressure acts as a stretching force, expanding the lung and decreasing alveolar pressure. The pressure at the mouth and nares is equal to atmospheric pressure, so as alveolar pressure decreases, a pressure gradient develops and gas flows through the airways into the alveoli. As the number of gas molecules in the alveoli increases, alveolar pressure increases until it equals atmospheric pressure, at which time gas flow, hence inspiration, ceases.

During exhalation, respiratory muscles relax, thoracic volume decreases, and pleural pressure increases. The elastic recoil of the lung and chest wall compresses the lung, increasing alveolar pressure. Since alveolar pressure is greater than atmospheric, gas flows out of the lung. As the number of gas molecules in the alveoli decreases, alveolar pressure decreases until it equals atmospheric pressure and gas flow, hence expiration, ceases.

Positive pressure ventilation. For positive pressure breathing, the total driving pressure is airway pressure minus atmospheric pressure (the pressure across the respiratory system [Figure 2]). During a positive pressure breath, the ventilator increases upper airway pressure above alveolar pressure, and gas flows into the alveoli. Alveolar pressure increases and provides the stretching force necessary to expand both the lung and chest wall. Because the lung pushes on the chest wall, pleural pressure is positive relative to atmospheric pressure. Gas flows into the lung until alveolar pressure equals airway pressure. Exhalation is passive and similar to that for a spontaneous breath.

Equation of motion and respiratory time constant. The mechanical behavior of the respiratory system over time can be described mathematically by the *equation of motion*. This equation states that the driving pressure, P(t), required to move gas in and out of the lung at a given time (t) during the respiratory cycle is the sum of the pressures required to overcome elastic [Pel(t)], resistive [Pr(t)], and inertance forces [Pi(t)]:

$$P(t) = Pel(t) + Pr(t) + Pi(t)$$

Now, Pel(t) = V(t)/C (the volume of the respiratory system at time [t] divided by the compliance) and

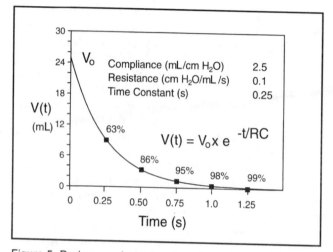

Figure 5: During passive exhalation, the volume of gas in the lung at any time (t) depends on the starting lung volume (V_o) and the product of resistance and compliance, the respiratory time constant. If exhalation proceeds for a time equal to 1 time constant, t = 1 x R x C (0.25 seconds in this example), this equation predicts that the volume of gas left in the lung will be roughly 0.37 x the initial volume (V_o), or the lung will be 63% empty. After 2 time constants, the lung will be 86% empty, and after 5 time constants, 99% empty. (Adapted from Hansen TN, Corbet AJ. In: Taeusch HW, et al, eds. *Schaffer and Avery's Diseases of the Newborn.* 5th ed. Philadelphia, WB Saunders, 1991.)

$Pr(t) = \dot{V}(t)$ x R (the rate of gas flow at time [t] times resistance). If we ignore inertance, the equation of motion simplifies to the first order differential equation:

$$P(t) = [V(t)/C] + [\dot{V}(t) \times R]$$

Special solutions to the equation of motion. While a general solution to the equation of motion is outside

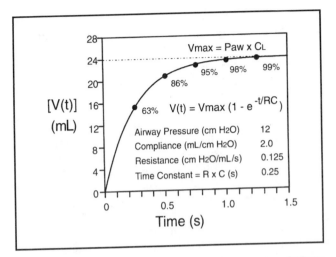

Figure 6: In this example, a constant airway pressure of 12 cm H₂O is applied to the airway. The equation predicts that at time equal to one time constant (0.25 seconds in this example), the lung will inflate to 63% of its maximum volume (Vmax), and if t = 5 x R x C the lung will inflate to 99% of Vmax.(Adapted from Hansen TN, Corbet AJ. In: Taeusch HW, et al, eds. *Schaffer and Avery's Diseases of the Newborn*. 5th ed. Philadelphia, WB Saunders, 1991.)

the scope of this handbook, there are several general solutions that are clinically useful:

Points of no gas flow. At end expiration and end inspiration, gas flow is zero, and the equation of motion reduces to $P(t) = V(t)/C$, ie, driving pressure is affected only by elastic forces. At all other times in the respiratory cycle, driving pressure must overcome both elastic and resistive forces.

Passive exhalation. The simplified equation of motion is useful in explaining the behavior of the respiratory system during passive exhalation. During passive exhalation, airway pressure [P(t)] equals atmospheric pressure, which equals 0, and the equation of motion has the simple solution:

$$V(t) = V_o \times e^{-t/R \times C} \text{ (see Figure 5).}$$

This solution allows us to calculate the volume of gas, V(t), remaining in the lung at any time (t) during a passive exhalation. V_o is the volume of gas in the lung at the beginning of exhalation, e is a constant roughly equal to 2.72, t is time, and R x C is the product of resistance and compliance. R x C has the units of time and is called the *respiratory time constant.*

The rate at which the lung empties during exhalation is determined by the time constant. If resistance or compliance decreases, the lung will empty more rapidly. Conversely, if resistance or compliance increases, the time constant increases and the lung empties more slowly. In particular, diseases that cause airway obstruction will increase resistance, increase the time constant, and cause the lung to empty more slowly.

During spontaneous or positive pressure ventilation, if the expiratory time is less than three time constants, the lung will not empty completely before the next inspiration. With each subsequent breath, additional gas will be trapped and the lung volume will increase. Lung overinflation secondary to this form of gas trapping often complicates the course of diseases that increase airway resistance and the respiratory time constant, such as bronchopulmonary dysplasia.

Interestingly, preterm infants may use this phenomenon to compensate for chest wall instability. As discussed earlier, because of a highly compliant chest wall, the preterm infant should have a decreased resting lung volume, FRC. However, when FRC is measured in spontaneously breathing preterm infants, it is often similar to that noted in term infants. This discrepancy occurs because the preterm infant breathes sufficiently fast to impinge upon expiration and traps enough gas to normalize FRC. Of course, during periodic breathing or apnea, this defense mechanism is lost and FRC falls.

Positive pressure inflation. Another special solution to the equation of motion occurs during inflation of the lung with a constant airway pressure, ie, the pressure in the lung over time [P(t)] equals airway pressure [Paw], which is constant. In this case,

$$V(t) = Vmax \; (1 - e^{-t/R \times C}) \; \text{(see Figure 6)}$$

Vmax is the maximum volume of lung inflation for a given airway pressure and equal to Paw x C_L. Therefore, our equation can be simplified to:

$$V(t) = Paw \times C_L \times (1 - e^{-t/R \times C})$$

According to this relationship, the maximum volume of gas that can be instilled into the lung during an infinitely long, positive pressure breath is limited by Paw x C_L. The rate at which the lung inflates to this volume is determined by the time constant, R x C. Increases or decreases in resistance will affect the rate of inflation but will not alter the ultimate lung volume. Changes in compliance, however, will affect the ultimate lung volume and the rate of inflation to that volume. The roles of resistance and compliance in lung inflation will be discussed in more detail in the sections on pulmonary function tests (Chapter 3) and positive pressure ventilation (Chapter 10).

By Thomas N. Hansen, MD

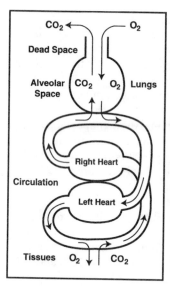

Figure 7: Oxygen uptake and delivery can be broken down into three components: (1) an intake and exhaust component—the lungs; (2) a delivery system—the circulation; and (3) an O_2 reservoir—the blood. Oxygen is extracted from the atmosphere by the lungs and delivered by the circulation to the tissues to support oxidative metabolism. Carbon dioxide generated by the tissues is transported back to the lung for excretion into the atmosphere. (Adapted from Hansen TN, Corbet AJ. In: Taeusch HW, et al, eds. *Schaffer and Avery's Diseases of the Newborn*. 5th ed. Philadelphia, WB Saunders, 1991.)

Oxygen Transport and Alveolar Ventilation

Individual cells take up oxygen (O_2) continuously from their environment to support oxidative metabolism and excrete carbon dioxide (CO_2), the byproduct of this metabolism. Evolution from single-celled organisms to multicellular organisms required the development of a complex system to allow cells to exchange gas with the environment (Figure 7).

Lungs: Alveolar Ventilation

The lung consists of a *preacinar* compartment containing the conducting airways to the level of the terminal bronchiole, and an *acinar* compartment containing respiratory bronchioles, alveolar ducts, and alveoli. The total volume of gas moving in and out of the lung with each breath is the *tidal volume*. The product of tidal volume and respiratory rate is the *minute ventilation*. The conducting airways do not ex-

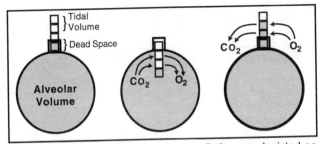

Figure 8: Alveolar and dead space ventilation are depicted as delivery of packets of atmospheric gas (white) to the lung. During inspiration, the packet of gas residing in the dead space (shaded) moves into the alveolar volume. This packet has gas tensions similar to alveolar gas and no net gas exchange occurs. As inspiration continues, packets of fresh gas move into the lung. These packets deliver O_2 to the alveolus and remove CO_2. Of the three packets of gas entering the lung from the atmosphere (the tidal volume), only two participate in gas exchange. The last packet of fresh gas occupies the dead space. At end inspiration, dead space gas tensions are identical to those of atmospheric gas. With expiration, the first packet of gas to leave the lung exits from the dead space and has gas tensions identical to atmospheric gas. As expiration continues, packets with gas tensions similar to those of alveolar gas exit the lung and the CO_2 tension of expired gas increases while its O_2 tension decreases. The last packet of expired gas fills the dead space so that at end exhalation the dead space gas tension is identical to that of alveolar gas. Measurement of end expired CO_2 and O_2 tensions provides a reasonable approximation of alveolar gas tensions.

change gas with blood and represent the *dead space volume* (Figure 8). The acinar compartment does exchange gas with the blood and represents the *alveolar volume* (Figure 8). Alveolar volume equals the tidal volume minus the dead space volume. Effective ventilation or *alveolar ventilation* is the product of the alveolar volume and the respiratory rate (Table 1).

Alveolar ventilation is intermittent, while tissue O_2 consumption and CO_2 production are continuous. Removal of O_2 from alveoli by the blood during expiration and addition

Table 2: Calculations of Alveolar Oxygen Tension, P_{AO_2}

Ventilation	Pa_{CO_2}	R	F_{IO_2}	BMP	P_{AO_2}
Hyperventilation	20	0.8	0.21	760	125
Normal	40	0.8	0.21	760	100
Hypoventilation	80	0.8	0.21	760	50
Hypoventilation	80	0.8	0.40	760	185
Normal	40	0.8	0.21	630	72

Using arterial CO_2 tension (Pa_{CO_2}) as an index of alveolar ventilation, alveolar O_2 tension (P_{AO_2}) can be calculated using a simplified alveolar-air equation:

$$P_{AO_2} = F_{IO_2} (BMP - P_{H_2O}) - Pa_{CO_2}/R.$$

F_{IO_2} is the fraction of inspired O_2, BMP is the barometric pressure (760 torr at sea level), P_{H_2O} is the partial pressure of water in alveolar gas (47 torr at 37°C) and R is the respiratory exchange ratio, usually 0.8 to 1.0, depending on the relative amount of fat versus carbohydrate being used as fuel. Since arterial O_2 tension is never greater than alveolar O_2 tension, this equation predicts the maximum arterial O_2 tension obtainable for any given F_{IO_2} and level of ventilation. Hyperventilation increases alveolar O_2 tension at any given F_{IO_2}. Hypoventilation decreases alveolar O_2 tension, hence arterial O_2 tension, and causes hypoxia when F_{IO_2} is 0.21 (room air). Supplemental O_2 (eg, $F_{IO_2} = 0.40$) relieves hypoxia secondary to hypoventilation. Ascending to an altitude of 5,000 ft (eg, Denver, CO) lowers the barometric pressure to 630 torr and decreases the alveolar oxygen tension and the arterial O_2 tension.

of CO_2 decreases alveolar O_2 tension and increases alveolar CO_2 tension. Arterial blood O_2 and CO_2 tensions are in equilibrium with those of alveolar gas and change similarly. Fortunately, the lung is provided with a buffer—the functional residual capacity—that is large (30 mL/kg body weight) compared with the tidal volume (5 to 7 mL/kg body weight). During expiration, this large buffer continues to provide O_2 to capillary blood and acts as a sump for CO_2 so that alveolar, hence arterial, gas tensions remain relatively constant over the respiratory cycle.

Alveolar ventilation is coupled to tissue O_2 consumption and CO_2 production. If alveolar ventilation increases so that O_2 uptake and CO_2 elimination by the lungs are greater than O_2 consumption and CO_2 production, the stores of O_2 in the lung and blood will increase and those of CO_2 will decrease. This is called *hyperventilation*. It will be reflected as an increased alveolar O_2 tension and decreased alveolar CO_2 tension. Conversely, a decrease in alveolar ventilation relative to O_2 consumption and CO_2 production is called *hypoventilation* and is reflected as a decreased alveolar O_2 tension and increased alveolar CO_2 tension. Generally, changes in arterial O_2 and CO_2 tensions are proportional to changes in alveolar O_2 and CO_2. Therefore, measurements of arterial CO_2 tension can be used to estimate changes in alveolar ventilation (Table 2).

The Circulation

Blood in the alveolar capillary bed equilibrates with alveolar gas, then returns to the heart via the pulmonary veins and left atrium, and is finally pumped to the tissues of the body by the left ventricle through the systemic arterial circulation (Figure 7). In the systemic capillary bed, O_2 is removed by the tissues to support oxidative metabolism. In the tissues, O_2 diffuses out of the capillaries, into the cells, and finally into the mitochondria along a gradient of partial pressures. The minimal O_2 tension necessary to maintain this diffusion gradient is the *critical O_2 tension*. End capillary Po_2 or mixed venous Po_2 helps maintain the driving pressure for tissue oxygenation, so mixed venous Po_2 must be maintained above the critical O_2 tension to ensure delivery of O_2 into the cells and mitochondria. Blood is then returned to the heart via the systemic venous circulation and right atrium and is then pumped to the lungs by the right ventricle through the pulmonary arteries. In the lungs, CO_2 is excreted and additional O_2 is taken up by the blood.

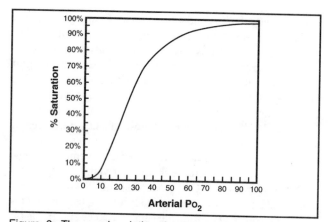

Figure 9: The graph relating the arterial O_2 tension and O_2 saturation is called the oxyhemoglobin dissociation curve. The flat upper portion of the curve ensures that blood passing through the lungs will be near fully saturated with O_2 over a wide range of alveolar O_2 tensions, while the steep middle portion of the curve allows a large volume of O_2 to be unloaded to the tissues while still maintaining mixed venous O_2 tension above the critical level for O_2 tension.

The Blood-Oxygen Reservoir

Oxygen content. Oxygen is transported in the blood bound to hemoglobin. One gram of hemoglobin can carry roughly 1.34 mL O_2. The binding of O_2 to hemoglobin is usually expressed as a percentage saturation, Sao_2, the ratio of oxygenated hemoglobin to total hemoglobin. The percentage saturation is a nonlinear function of the Pao_2 (Figure 9).

The position of the oxyhemoglobin dissociation curve is affected by changes in type of hemoglobin, pH, temperature, and concentrations of 2,3-diphosphoglycerate (2,3-DPG). Fetal hemoglobin binds O_2 more avidly than does adult hemoglobin and tends to shift the curve to the left. As a result, the Pao_2 at which hemoglobin is 50% saturated (P_{50}) is decreased. This shift benefits the fetus since it favors O_2 uptake at the low O_2 tensions in the placenta. However, in the newborn,

Table 3: Factors Affecting the Position of the Oxyhemoglobin Dissociation Curve

Shift Curve to the Left and ⇓ P50	Shift Curve to the Right and ⇑ P50
(Impair Oxygen Delivery)	*(Improve Oxygen Delivery)*
• Alkalosis	• Acidosis
• ⇓ Temperature	• ⇑ Temperature
• ⇓ 2,3-DPG concentrations	• ⇑ 2,3-DPG concentrations
• ⇑ Fetal hemoglobin	• ⇑ Adult hemoglobin

this left shift may impair O_2 delivery to the tissues because mixed venous O_2 tension, therefore, the tissue Po_2 favoring diffusion of O_2 into cells, is decreased (Table 3). During the first months after birth, the oxyhemoglobin dissociation curve begins to shift to the right, and between 4 and 6 months of age it is similar to that of the adult.

A small amount of O_2 is also carried dissolved in plasma (0.003 mL for each torr of Pao_2). The volume of dissolved O_2 is linearly related to the Pao_2 (Figure 10).

Oxygen delivery. Oxygen delivery to the tissues is the product of arterial oxygen content and cardiac output, and it is directly affected by changes in Pao_2, hemoglobin concentration [Hb], and cardiac output. A decrease in any one of these components can be offset to some extent by increases in the others (Figure 11).

Oxygen consumption is equal to the cardiac output times the difference between arterial O_2 content and venous O_2 content. Oxygen consumption can be affected by both O_2 deliv-

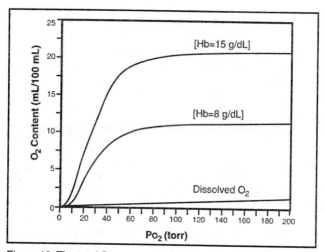

Figure 10: The total O₂ content of blood is the sum of the O₂ bound to hemoglobin (1.34 mL O_2/g Hb x [Hb] x Sao_2) plus the dissolved O_2 (0.003 mL O_2/torr x Pao_2), where [Hb] is the hemoglobin concentration of blood in g/dL. The relationship between Po_2 and O_2 content is curvilinear because of the shape of the oxyhemoglobin dissociation curve. A change in Po_2 in the steep part of the curve from 40 to 80 torr results in a large change in content, while a large change in Pao_2 on the flat part of the curve from 80 to 400 torr has much less effect. Note the profound effect of changes in [Hb] and the small effect of changes in dissolved O_2 on O_2 content.

ery and by the ability of the tissues to extract O_2 from blood. The difference between arterial O_2 content and venous O_2 content is a measure of effectiveness of O_2 delivery to tissues. *An increase in the gradient between arterial and venous O_2 contents infers that delivery is inadequate and that the tissues are increasing extraction to maintain O_2 consumption.* The ability to lower the mixed venous O_2 tension and increase extraction is limited, since a minimum gradient of oxygen tension must be maintained to facilitate diffusion of oxygen into cells and mitochondria. If mixed venous O_2 tension falls too low, O_2 delivery to mitochondria will be com-

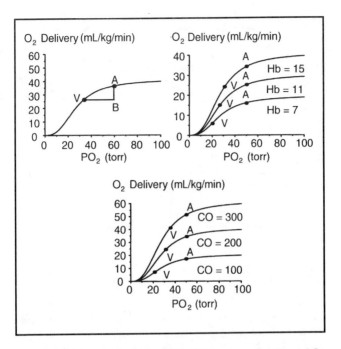

Figure 11: At top left is a plot of O_2 delivery as a function of O_2 tension for a fixed cardiac output of 200 mL/kg/min, a hemoglobin concentration of 15 g/dL, and an O_2 consumption of 10 mL/kg/min. At the arterial point A, an arterial O_2 tension of 60 torr results in an O_2 delivery to the tissues of nearly 35 mL/kg/min. If 10 mL/kg/min of O_2 is removed by the tissues, then the 'delivery of O_2' back to the heart from the tissues is roughly 25 mL/kg/min. This removal of O_2 decreases the O_2 tension at the venous point (V) to roughly 30 torr. In the top right figure, O_2 delivery is plotted as a function of O_2 tension for a constant cardiac output (200 mL/kg/min) and varying hemoglobin (g/dL) concentrations. On the bottom figure, O_2 delivery is plotted at a constant hemoglobin concentration and varying cardiac outputs (mL/kg/min). At arterial O_2 tensions over 50 torr, hemoglobin concentration and cardiac output have the most profound effects on O_2 delivery. Also note that at a constant arterial O_2 tension (A), as O_2 delivery decreases, the O_2 tension of venous blood (V) decreases.

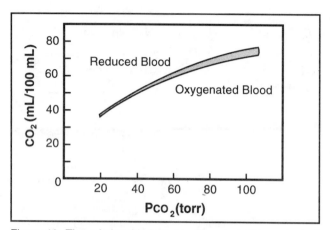

Figure 12: The relationship between P_{CO_2} and CO_2 content of blood is nearly linear. Mixed venous P_{CO_2} is about 6 torr higher than arterial P_{CO_2}. The CO_2 content of reduced blood is greater than that of oxygenated blood.

promised and O_2 consumption will decrease as the cell switches from aerobic to anaerobic metabolism. Anaerobic metabolism is much less efficient, generating only 2 mol of adenosine triphosphate (ATP)/mol glucose compared with 38 mol of ATP/mol glucose for aerobic metabolism. This inefficiency results in ATP depletion and ultimate cell death. In addition, anaerobic metabolism generates two molecules of lactic acid for every molecule of glucose metabolized, resulting in tissue lactic acidosis. *Therefore, the appearance of significant amounts of lactic acid in blood (> 3 mmol/L) is indicative of inadequate O_2 delivery to the cellular mitochondria.*

Carbon Dioxide Transport

Oxygen transport evolved to optimize oxygen-carrying capacity in room air. Carbon dioxide transport, however, evolved so that large amounts could be excreted continuously from high body concentrations to low atmospheric concentrations. Carbon dioxide can be carried by the body in several forms: dissolved in plasma, as bicarbonate in equilibrium with dissolved CO_2, or carried by amino acid groups in hemoglobin. The largest fraction of CO_2 is in the form of plasma or red cell bicarbonate. Carbon dioxide is 20 times more soluble in blood than oxygen, and its dissociation curve is nearly linear over physiologic ranges. As a result, large amounts of CO_2 can be carried in blood and removed from the body with relatively small changes in blood CO_2 tension (Figure 12).

Carbon dioxide and oxygen interact in the blood to enhance each other's loading and unloading capabilities where concentration extremes exist. The binding of CO_2 to hemoglobin in the tissues augments unloading of oxygen from capillary blood—the *Bohr effect*. On the other hand, the binding of oxygen to hemoglobin in the alveolar capillary bed augments CO_2 unloading from capillary blood into the alveolar space—the *Haldane effect*.
By Michael R. Gomez, MD, and Thomas N. Hansen, MD

Ventilation-Perfusion Relationships

The four causes of arterial hypoxemia in infants are hypoventilation, diffusion block, ventilation-perfusion mismatch, and right-to-left shunt (Table 4). Hypoxemia secondary to hypoventilation is discussed in the previous section. Hypoxemia secondary to diffusion block is virtually nonexistent in the newborn and will not be addressed further. Therefore, the rest of this chapter will focus on hypoxemia secondary to ventilation-perfusion mismatch (Figure 13) and right-to-left shunt.

Ventilation-Perfusion Mismatch
Distribution of Ventilation and Alveolar Gas Tensions

In the simplest form of ventilation-perfusion ($\dot{V}_A/\dot{Q}$) mismatch, the lung is divided into two ventilatory compartments. One is normal or *well ventilated*, while the other is abnormal secondary to parenchymal lung disease and is *poorly ventilated*.

Table 4: Cause of Hypoxemia

Cause of Hypoxemia	Pa_{CO_2}	Hypoxemia Relieved by ⇑ F_{IO_2}
Hypoventilation	⇑	Yes
Diffusion Block	⇒	Yes
Ventilation-Perfusion Mismatch	⇒ ⇓	Yes
Right-to-Left Shunt	⇒ ⇓	No

The well-ventilated compartment receives a disproportionate share of each tidal volume, and the minute ventilation serves to exchange gas predominantly with this compartment. If blood flow to each compartment is equal, the well-ventilated compartment is ventilated out of proportion to its level of perfusion. It has a high ventilation-to-perfusion ratio ($\dot{V}_A/\dot{Q}$ >1) and is analogous to a single hyperventilated lung unit. It has a low alveolar CO_2 tension (P_{CO_2}) and a high alveolar O_2 tension (P_{O_2}) (see *Oxygen Transport and Alveolar Ventilation* section, this chapter). The poorly ventilated compartment is perfused out of proportion to its level of ventilation and has a low ventilation-to-perfusion ratio ($\dot{V}_A/\dot{Q}$ <1). It is hypoventilated relative to its level of perfusion and has a high alveolar CO_2 tension and low alveolar O_2 tension.

Effects of $\dot{V}_A/\dot{Q}$ Mismatch on Blood Gas Tensions

Well-ventilated compartment. In the capillary bed of the *well-ventilated compartment*, mixed venous blood equilibrates with alveolar gas, and its O_2 tension increases and CO_2 tension decreases. The increased O_2 tension increases O_2 saturation and content. Blood flowing through this compartment is termed *idealized capillary blood*.

Poorly ventilated compartment. In the capillary bed of the *poorly ventilated compartment*, mixed venous blood also

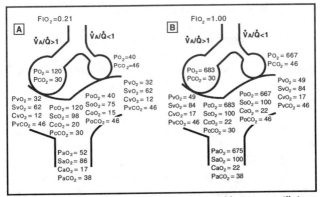

Figure 13: Both A and B depict a lung with two ventilatory compartments—one normal ($\dot{V}_A/\dot{Q}$ >1) and the other severely underventilated ($\dot{V}_A/\dot{Q}$ <1). In Figure A, the F_{IO_2} is room air and in B it is 100% O_2. Barometric pressure is 760 mm Hg, respiratory exchange ratio is 1.0, cardiac output is 200 mL/kg/min, hemoglobin concentration is 15 g/dL, and O_2 consumption is 10 mL/kg/min. In each figure, 50% of the total blood flow goes past each compartment. The abbreviations are defined below. See text for discussion.

Measurement	Units	Compartment			
		Mixed Venous	Ideal Capillary	Poorly Ventilated	Mixed Arterial
O_2 Tension	mm Hg	PvO_2	PcO_2	PoO_2	PaO_2
O_2 Saturation	%	SvO_2	ScO_2	SoO_2	SaO_2
O_2 Content	mL O_2/100 mL blood	CvO_2	CcO_2	CoO_2	CaO_2
CO_2 Tension	mm Hg	$PvCO_2$	$PcCO_2$	$PoCO_2$	$PaCO_2$

equilibrates with alveolar gas. However, alveolar gas tensions are similar to those of mixed venous blood, so O_2 tension increases only slightly, while CO_2 tension remains virtually unchanged. In fact, mixed venous gas tensions form the limits for alveolar gas tensions in this compartment. Alveolar O_2 tension cannot be lower than the O_2 tension of mixed venous blood, nor can alveolar CO_2 tension be higher than the CO_2 tension of mixed venous blood, no matter how severely ventilation is impaired.

Mixed arterial O_2 tension. Blood from the well-ventilated and poorly ventilated compartments combines to form *mixed arterial blood*. The O_2 content of mixed arterial blood is determined by the O_2 content and the relative blood flow through each compartment. Because the oxyhemoglobin dissociation curve is nonlinear, the O_2 content of mixed arterial blood must be calculated before calculating mixed arterial O_2 tension. Mixed arterial O_2 content is equal to the fraction of blood flowing past normal alveoli times its O_2 content plus the fraction of blood flowing past poorly ventilated alveoli times its O_2 content. Mixed arterial Po_2 is determined from plots of arterial O_2 tension vs content and O_2 saturation from the oxyhemoglobin dissociation curve (see *Oxygen Transport and Alveolar Ventilation* section, this chapter).

Mixed arterial CO_2 tension. Since the plot of blood CO_2 tension vs CO_2 content is roughly linear, mixed arterial CO_2 tension can be calculated from the capillary CO_2 tensions and relative blood flows of each compartment.

Mixed venous O_2 tension. Since $\dot{V}_A/\dot{Q}$ mismatch decreases arterial O_2 content, it must also decrease mixed venous O_2 content, if O_2 consumption and cardiac output remain constant (see *Oxygen Transport and Alveolar Ventilation* section, this chapter). In Figure 13, mixed venous oxygen content can be calculated from O_2 consumption and calculated O_2 delivery.

Venous admixture. *In infants with $\dot{V}_A/\dot{Q}$ mismatch, the severity of hypoxemia is determined by the relative proportion of blood flow through the open, poorly ventilated lung compartment.* The contribution of $\dot{V}_A/\dot{Q}$ mismatch to arterial hypoxemia can be calculated as the venous admixture. The venous admixture is that fraction of mixed venous return that is not oxygenated above mixed venous levels upon passing through the lung. It is calculated using the values for ideal pulmonary capillary O_2 content (CcO_2), mixed arterial O_2 content (CaO_2), and mixed venous O_2 content (CvO_2):

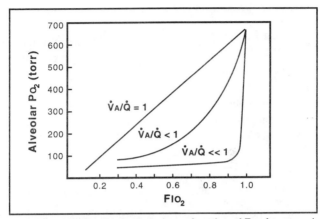

Figure 14: Alveolar Po_2 is plotted as a function of Fio_2 for normal alveoli $\dot{V}_A/\dot{Q} = 1$ and for alveoli that are progressively underventilated with respect to their perfusion, $\dot{V}_A/\dot{Q} < 1$. As ventilation decreases relative to perfusion, more O_2 is removed from the alveolus by the blood than can be replaced by alveolar ventilation, and the alveolar Po_2 decreases. For severely underventilated units, $\dot{V}_A/\dot{Q} < 1$, alveolar Po_2 increases only when Fio_2 approaches 1.00. The dramatic increase in alveolar Po_2 occurs because of nitrogen washout (Table 5). (Adapted from Hansen TN, Corbet AJ. In: Taeusch HW, et al, eds. *Schaffer and Avery's Diseases of the Newborn.* 5th ed. Philadelphia, WB Saunders, 1991.)

Venous admixture = $[(CcO_2 - CaO_2)/(CcO_2 - CvO_2)] \times 100\%$. In the example in Figure 13A, the venous admixture is 38%.

Effect of Increased Fio_2 on Venous Admixture

Because the poorly ventilated alveoli are open to the airway, increasing the inspired O_2 tension should increase their alveolar Po_2 (Figure 14). In Figure 13B, increasing Fio_2 to 1.00 dramatically increases the Po_2 in the open but poorly ventilated lung units. The O_2 content of the blood perfusing these units increases 30%, while the O_2 content of the blood perfusing the well-ventilated units increases only 10%. As a result, the O_2 content of mixed arterial blood increases. The calculated venous admixture is now near zero. Note that most of the increase in mixed arterial O_2 content was the result of increased O_2 content in the open but poorly ventilated alveoli. This example demonstrates an important concept. *The cause of hypoxemia in infants with $\dot{V}_A/\dot{Q}$ mismatch is perfusion of poorly ventilated but open alveoli. The only way to increase the arterial P_{O_2} in these infants is to increase the P_{O_2} in these poorly ventilated alveoli (Table 5).*

Right-to-Left Shunt

Blood that flows from the venous circulation (the right side of the circulation) to the arterial circulation (the left side of the circulation) without flowing past an open lung unit results in a *right-to-left shunt*. There are three pathways through which right-to-left shunt may occur:

- through the lung, past areas of atelectasis or through vessels that develop before alveoli form;

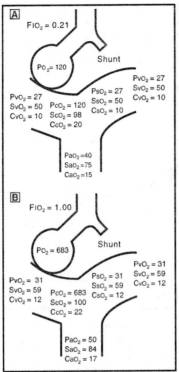

Figure 15: A and B each depict a lung with a well-ventilated compartment and right-to-left shunt. In A, the $FIO_2 = 0.21$ and in B the $FIO_2 = 1.00$. The modifier 's' refers to blood flowing through the shunt. In both figures, half of the mixed venous return flows through the shunt and half past normal lung units. The other abbreviations and assumptions are the same as for Figure 13.

- through persistent fetal circulatory pathways such as the foramen ovale or ductus arteriosus;
- through abnormal structures resulting from congenital abnormalities of the heart and great vessels.

Right-to-left shunt represents a special case of $\dot{V}A/\dot{Q}$ mismatch where ventilation equals zero, hence $\dot{V}A/\dot{Q} = 0$ (Figure 15).

Effects of Shunt on Mixed Arterial Blood Gas Tensions

Mixed arterial O_2 tension. In infants with right-to-left shunt (Figure 15), mixed venous blood returns to the lung poorly oxygenated. A portion of this blood flows past normal alveoli where it equilibrates with alveolar gas and be-

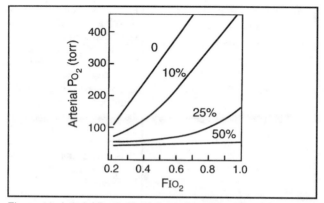

Figure 16: Arterial P_{O_2} is plotted as a function of F_{IO_2} for a variety of right-to-left shunts. When the total right-to-left shunt exceeds 50%, there is little effect of increasing F_{IO_2} on arterial P_{O_2}. (Adapted from Benator SR, et al: *Br J Anaesth* 1973;45:722.)

comes well oxygenated *(ideal capillary blood)*. The remainder, the true right-to-left shunt, flows from the mixed venous to the arterial circulation without passing an open lung unit and remains poorly oxygenated *(shunt blood)*. These two streams of blood mix before returning to the heart. The O_2 content of this mixed arterial blood is determined both by the O_2 content and relative blood flows through each compartment. The effects of right-to-left shunt on mixed arterial O_2 content, O_2 saturation, and O_2 tension can be calculated as described in the section on $\dot{V}_A/\dot{Q}$ mismatch. Since shunt decreases arterial O_2 content, it also decreases mixed venous O_2 content if O_2 consumption and cardiac output remain constant.

Mixed arterial CO_2 tension. Mixed arterial CO_2 tension is calculated as described for $\dot{V}_A/\dot{Q}$ mismatch. The normal lung compartment is relatively hyperventilated, while the ventilation in the shunt compartment equals zero.

Shunt equation. Using the values for ideal pulmonary capillary O_2 content (CcO_2), mixed arterial O_2 content (CaO_2), and mixed venous O_2 content (CvO_2), we can calculate the percentage for the shunt: $[(CcO_2 - CaO_2)/(CcO_2 - CvO_2)] \times 100\%$. In the example in Figure 15 the shunt is 50%.

Effect of Increased F$_{IO_2}$ on Right-to-Left Shunt

Arterial hypoxemia secondary to right-to-left shunt cannot be completely relieved by administration of supplemental O_2 (Figure 15B). Increasing F$_{IO_2}$ increases the O_2 content of blood flowing through the normally ventilated compartment but does not affect the O_2 content of the blood flowing through the shunt. While mixed arterial O_2 tension will increase slightly because of the small increase in O_2 content of blood flowing past normal alveoli, this increase is relatively small compared to that noted with $\dot{V}A/\dot{Q}$ mismatch (Figure 13B). *More importantly, the calculated shunt remains 50%.* The effects of right-to-left shunt on arterial O_2 tension are shown graphically in Figure 16.

Combination $\dot{V}A/\dot{Q}$ Mismatch and Right-to-Left Shunt Disorders

In most clinical conditions, hypoxemia is a result of a combination of $\dot{V}A/\dot{Q}$ mismatch and right-to-left shunt (Figure 17). Well-oxygenated blood flowing past well-ventilated alveoli mixes with poorly oxygenated blood flowing past open poorly ventilated alveoli and blood flowing through the right-to-left shunt. The mixed arterial O_2 content depends on both the O_2 content and the relative amounts of blood flowing through each of these three compartments. The *venous admixture* is that fraction of blood returning to the left side of the heart that is not oxygenated above mixed venous O_2 content. For values of F$_{IO_2}$ <1.00, blood flowing past poorly ventilated alveoli and blood flowing through the right-to-left shunt both contribute to the venous admixture. When F$_{IO_2}$ equals 1.00, any contribution to the venous admixture from open, poorly ventilated alveoli disappears (Figure 13B). *Therefore, when F$_{IO_2}$ = 1.00, the size of the venous admixture is determined only by the size of the right-to-left shunt, ie, percent venous admixture = percent shunt.* This phenom-

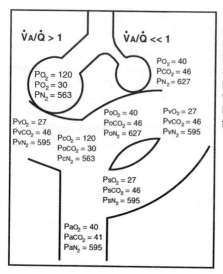

Figure 17: In this example of a combination disorder, hypoxemia is the result of perfusion of poorly ventilated alveoli and right-to-left shunt. See text for discussion.

enon is the basis for the hyperoxia test. If an infant breathes 100% O_2, any contribution from the perfusion of poorly ventilated alveoli to arterial hypoxemia is abolished and any remaining hypoxemia must be the result of right-to-left shunt. Failure to increase arterial O_2 content, saturation, or tension while breathing 100% O_2 is strongly suggestive of anatomic right-to-left shunt and congenital heart disease.

Arterial-Alveolar Gas Tension Gradients

In the simple one-compartment model of the lung used to describe alveolar ventilation, it was assumed that capillary blood equilibrated completely with alveolar gas so that arterial blood gas tensions were identical to alveolar gas tensions. This is also true for the multicompartment lung, provided that all compartments are equally well ventilated and well perfused, ie, all have $\dot{V}_A/\dot{Q} = 1$. In the face of ventilation and perfusion mismatch, however, alveolar gas tensions are not equal to arterial gas tensions (Figure 17).

Table 6: Calculation of Alveolar and Mixed Arterial Gradients from the Example in Figure 17

	Alveolar (mm Hg)	Mixed Arterial (mm Hg)	Gradient (mm Hg)
O_2	120	40	A-aDO_2=80
CO_2	30	41	a-ADCO_2=11
N_2	563	595	a-ADN_2=32
A-a: Alveolar to arterial; a-A: Arterial to alveolar			

In lungs with unequal ventilation, most of each tidal volume enters and leaves the well-ventilated compartment ($\dot{V}A/\dot{Q} >1$). Therefore, the composition of end tidal expired gas is determined predominantly by the alveolar gas composition in the well-ventilated compartment (Table 6 and Figure 17). The three commonly used alveolar-arterial gas gradients, A-aDO_2, a-ADCO_2, and a-ADN_2, are calculated in Table 6.

A-aDO_2. The alveolar to arterial gradient for O_2 is used to estimate the severity of arterial hypoxemia. It is increased both by increased perfusion of poorly ventilated alveoli and by increased blood flow through the right-to-left shunt. In patients breathing pure O_2, the A-aDO_2 is determined solely by the size of the right-to-left shunt. In patients with a right-to-left shunt, the A-aDO_2 increases with increasing FIO_2 and as such is a poor estimate of lung disease severity (Figure 16).

a-ADCO_2. The arterial to alveolar gradient for CO_2 arises because some alveoli are ventilated out of proportion to their perfusion. These hyperventilated alveoli with low alveolar CO_2 tensions determine the CO_2 tensions of end tidal gas. The CO_2 tension of mixed arterial blood is determined by the CO_2 tensions in all lung compartments. An increased a-ADCO_2 implies that some alveoli are ventilated out of proportion to their perfusion *(physiologic dead space)*, and as such it is an estimate of wasted ventilation.

a-AD$_{N_2}$. The arterial to alveolar gradient for N_2 is the result of perfusion of open but poorly ventilated alveoli. Alveolar or end-tidal N_2 tension is determined by the N_2 tension in well-ventilated lung units. Mixed arterial N_2 tension is determined by the N_2 tension in blood from all lung compartments. In severely underventilated alveoli, the alveolar O_2 tension is reduced because O_2 extraction by blood exceeds its replacement by alveolar ventilation. Alveolar P_{CO_2} is fixed by mixed venous P_{CO_2}, and P_{H_2O} is determined by body temperature. If the alveolus is open to the airway, the sum of partial pressures must equal 760 mm Hg. As a result, alveolar N_2 tension increases. The N_2 tension of blood perfusing these alveoli also increases; and, when it mixes with blood from both the well-ventilated compartment and from the right-to-left shunt, mixed arterial N_2 tension increases. N_2 is neither produced nor consumed in the tissues, so mixed arterial N_2 tension is equal to mixed venous N_2 tension. Therefore, the N_2 tension of blood from the right-to-left shunt is equal to that of mixed venous blood (mixed arterial N_2 tension) and the a-AD$_{N_2}$ is not affected by the size of the right-to-left shunt. *The a-AD$_{N_2}$ only increases if the volume of blood flow past open but poorly ventilated alveoli increases. As a result, the a-AD$_{N_2}$ is a measure of their contribution to the venous admixture.*
By Thomas N. Hansen, MD, and James M. Adams, MD

Lung and Heart Interaction

Pleural Pressure

The lungs, heart, and great vessels all share the thoracic cavity. As a result, changes in pleural pressure (Ppl) directly affect the heart and great vessels as well as the lungs (Figure 18).

Decreased Ppl reduces the pressure surrounding the heart and literally sucks blood from systemic veins into the right atrium, increasing venous return and right ventricular output.

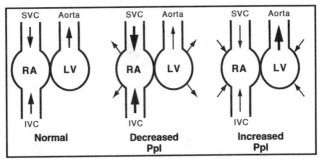

Figure 18: Effects of pleural pressure on blood return to the right atrium (RA) via the superior vena cava (SVC) and inferior vena cava (IVC) and ejection of blood from the left ventricle (LV) into the aorta.

Table 7: Conditions Causing Sustained Increases in Pleural Pressure	
Lung Overinflation	**Distention of the Pleural Space**
Overzealous mechanical ventilation	Pneumothorax
Pulmonary interstitial emphysema	Chylothorax
Cystic lung diseases	Pleural effusion

However, the same decrease in Ppl impedes left ventricular contraction and impairs left ventricular output. In infants with hyaline membrane disease, Ppl decreases markedly with inspiration. Consequently, left ventricular stroke volume and systolic blood pressure decrease with inspiration. If blood pressure is continuously monitored via an indwelling arterial catheter, this 'fluctuating blood pressure' is very apparent. The magnitude of the decrease in systolic blood pressure with inspiration is proportional to the decrease in Ppl, hence it is a marker of the severity of the lung disease.

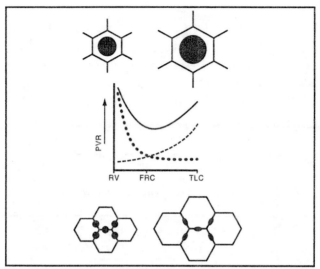

Figure 19: There are two types of blood vessels (shaded circles) in the lung: (1) Extra-alveolar vessels (top) that course in the extra-alveolar interstitium with airways and lymphatics; and (2) intra-alveolar vessels (bottom) that course through the intra-alveolar septa. During lung inflation, mechanical forces dilate extra-alveolar vessels, while the intra-alveolar vessels are compressed within the alveolar walls. Therefore, vascular resistance (PVR) of extra-alveolar vessels decreases with lung inflation (dotted line), while that of intra-alveolar vessels increases (dashed line). The net result is that total pulmonary vascular resistance (solid line) is lowest at resting lung volume, FRC, and increases at lung volumes above or below FRC (graph in middle). (Adapted from Hansen TN, Corbet AJ. In: Taeusch HW, et al, eds. *Schaffer and Avery's Diseases of the Newborn*. 5th ed. Philadelphia, WB Saunders, 1991.)

Increased Ppl compresses the heart, impairs venous return, and decreases right ventricular output. Sustained increases in Ppl may occur secondarily to lung overinflation or space-occupying lesions of the pleura (Table 7).

Conversely, cyclical increases in Ppl also compress the left ventricle, transiently augmenting ventricular systole and increasing left ventricular output. This phenomenon explains the maintenance of the circulation during external cardiac massage.

Alveolar Volume

Lung inflation directly affects the resistance to blood flow across the lung (Figure 19). Alveolar overdistention secondary to gas trapping or overzealous mechanical ventilation compresses intra-alveolar vessels and markedly increases pulmonary vascular resistance. The increase in resistance, coupled with the decrease in systemic venous return that occurs if pleural pressure becomes positive, results in severe hypotension. In addition, the compression of vessels in alveolar walls will increase pulmonary vascular resistance and shunt blood away from the lung through fetal pathways (see *PPHN*, Chapter 4, and $\dot{V}_A/\dot{Q}$ *Mismatch*, this chapter), resulting in hypoxia refractory to increases in F_{IO_2}.

By Kerry D. Stewart, MD, and Thomas N. Hansen, MD

Surfactant

Surface Tension

The internal surface area of the human lung occupies approximately 1 m²/kg body weight. This surface is lined by a layer of fluid that creates an air-liquid interface. At this interface, water molecules are attracted to other water molecules in the liquid phase. This attraction minimizes the surface area exposed to the air phase. These same forces cause water to form beads on a glass surface. In the lung, the net result is a tendency of alveoli to collapse according to the Pierre Simon de Laplace equation: $P = 2 \times T/R$, where P is the pressure needed to resist collapse, T is the surface tension, and R is the radius of the alveolus. According to this equation, as surface tension increases, the amount of pressure needed to overcome surface tension forces also increases. Calculations suggest that if the alveoli were lined only by water, it would take pressures exceeding 55 cm H_2O to inflate the lungs. Furthermore, since the pressure needed to resist collapse is inversely proportional to the radius, the Laplace equation predicts that

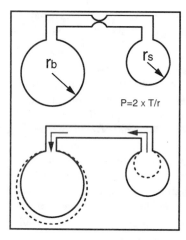

Figure 20: Two bubbles of unequal size are connected by a tube. When the tube is closed (top), there is no gas flow. When the tube is open (bottom), according to the Laplace equation, the pressure will be greater in the smaller bubble (radius r_s) than in the large bubble (radius r_b). As a result, gas will flow from the small bubble into the large bubble.

$P = 2 \times T/r$

small alveoli would tend to empty into large alveoli and that the lung would proceed to complete collapse at end exhalation (Figure 20). Of course, individuals breathe using far less inflation pressure because of the presence in the alveolar lining liquid of *surfactant*, which lowers surface tension forces. This substance is pulmonary *surfactant*.

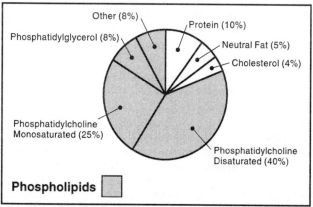

Figure 21: The composition of surfactant.

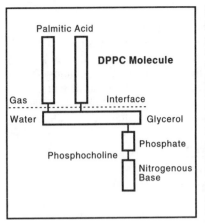

Figure 22: DPPC consists of two molecules of palmitic acid and one molecule of phosphocholine attached to a glycerol backbone. DPPC has a hydrophobic end (fatty acids) and hydrophilic end (nitrogenous base) and aligns itself in the air-liquid interface with the hydrophobic end in the gas phase and the hydrophilic end in the water phase.

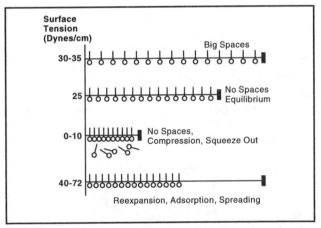

Figure 23: At equilibrium, surfactant displaces water molecules from the surface and lowers the surface tension from 72 dynes/cm to roughly 25 dynes/cm. At low lung volumes DPPC resists compression and lowers surface tension to near zero, further ensuring alveolar stability. During compression of the surface, some surfactant molecules are squeezed out into the bulk phase. With reexpansion of the lung, any lag in returning these molecules to the surface will result in increased surface tension.

Surfactant Function

Surfactant is produced in type II alveolar epithelial cells. It is composed of phospholipid with small amounts of neutral fat, cholesterol, and protein (Figure 21). The primary active molecule is saturated dipalmitoyl phosphatidylcholine (DPPC) (Figure 22). Other components of surfactant, including unsaturated phosphatidylcholine and phosphatidylglycerol, are important in making surfactant more fluid and facilitating respreading. Surfactant lowers surface tension by adsorbing to the surface and displacing water molecules (Figure 23).

Surfactant Proteins

There are four different proteins associated with the pulmonary surfactant: SP-A, SP-B, SP-C, and SP-D.

SP-A is the most abundant of the surfactant proteins, constituting nearly 5% by weight of the surfactant. It is a water-soluble protein composed of 228 amino acids in its monomeric state. The active protein consists of 18 monomeric units. SP-A reacts with SP-B, calcium, and surfactant to form *tubular myelin*, a latticelike network of lipoprotein that is highly surface active and increases adsorption of the surfactant lipids to the air-liquid interface. SP-A plays a role in surfactant recycling by enhancing the phospholipid uptake by alveolar type II cells and inhibiting phospholipid secretion. Finally, SP-A plays a role in host defense in the lung.

SP-B is a hydrophobic protein whose 381 amino acid preprotein is proteolytically processed in the cell to a 79 amino acid active protein. It is important in the formation of tubular myelin and relatively small amounts (<1% by weight) dramatically alter spreading and adsorption of the surfactant. SP-B also enhances uptake of surfactant by alveolar type II cells and may play a role in recycling of surfactant. The importance of SP-B in the lung has recently been underscored from the case reports of several term infants with congenital SP-B deficiency. These infants presented with severe respiratory distress progressing to respiratory failure. Treatment consisted of prolonged extracorporeal membrane oxygenation (ECMO) support followed by lung transplantation.

SP-C is a hydrophobic protein that constitutes roughly 0.4% of the surfactant by weight. Its 197 amino acid precursor protein is processed in the cell to a 35-36 amino acid active protein. It enhances the rate of adsorption and spreading of the surfactant. In addition, it enhances uptake of phospholipid vesicles by type II cells and may also play a role in surfactant recycling.

SP-D is the most recent of the surfactant proteins to be described. It constitutes only 0.2% by weight of the surfactant and is similar to SP-A in structure. Its functions are most likely related to host defense mechanisms in the lung.

Surfactant Synthesis

DPPC and other lipids are synthesized in the smooth endoplasmic reticulum of the type II alveolar epithelial cell. The lipids are transported in vesicles along microtubules and are stored in the lamellar bodies. The surfactant proteins are synthesized outside the rough endoplasmic reticulum, glycosylated in the Golgi apparatus, and then incorporated into the lamellar bodies. Lung inflation activates beta receptors in the type II cells to mobilize intracellular calcium, and the contents of the lamellar bodies are excreted into the air space. The secreted lipoprotein is converted into tubular myelin, a specialized form of surfactant, that rapidly moves to the surface of the air-liquid interface. After secretion, surfactant phospholipids can be taken back up into the type II cells by endocytosis and rapidly converted back into lamellar bodies for resecretion. The turnover time for surfactant is roughly 10 hours.

Type II alveolar epithelial cells begin to appear in the lung between 20 and 24 weeks' gestation. DPPC can be measured in whole lung extracts about this time and increases after 24 weeks. The presence of surfactant in the alveolar fluid lags considerably behind its appearance in lung tissue. Corticosteroids and thyroid hormone increase the rate of synthesis

Table 8: Risk of HMD as a Function of Amniotic Fluid Lecithin/Sphingo-myelin Ratio (L/S) and Phosphatidylglycerol (PG)

Amniotic Fluid	Risk of HMD
L/S >2.0 *	<0.5%
L/S <1.0	100%
L/S 1.0 to 2.0	⇓ as L/S ⇑
PG present	<0.5%
L/S <2.0; PG absent	>80%
L/S >2.0; PG present	0

*In pregnancies complicated by diabetes or Rh isoimmunization, the risk of HMD with an L/S between 2 and 3 is roughly 13%.

by increasing both the rate of transcription and the synthesis of important rate-limiting enzymes.

The lung of the fetus is not collapsed, but is filled with a fluid that is secreted by cells of the alveolar/airway epithelium. Throughout the latter part of gestation, this fluid wells up through the trachea and is either swallowed or excreted into the amniotic cavity. As a result, the fetal lung fluid contributes to the overall amniotic fluid volume and composition. Any substances, such as surfactant, secreted into the fetal alveolar space will eventually wind up in the amniotic fluid. It is possible to estimate fetal lung maturity by measuring the concentration of components of the pulmonary surfactant in the amniotic fluid. Usually, this is done by measuring the concentration of phosphatidylcholine or lecithin on samples of amniotic fluid obtained at amniocentesis. Because changes in amniotic fluid volume can change the lecithin concentration, these measurements are compared to the concentration of sphingomyelin, which remains relatively constant during gestation. The L/S ratio increases slowly between 24 and 32 weeks' gestation to about 1 and then surges at 34 to 35 weeks' gestation to greater than 2. Phosphatidylglycerol secretion into the lung, hence into amniotic fluid, also increases dramatically after 35 weeks' gestation. Its presence or absence also reflects lung maturity.

The risk of hyaline membrane disease (HMD) can be predicted from individual studies or combinations of studies as depicted in Table 8.

An adequate amount of surfactant in the air-liquid interface is crucial to alveolar stability. Surfactant deficiency results from an imbalance between the production and utilization of surfactant. Since surfactant production and secretion are developmentally regulated processes, the most common cause of deficiency is early or preterm delivery (see *Hyaline Membrane Disease*, Chapter 4).

By Alicia A. Moïse, MD, and Thomas N. Hansen, MD

Suggested Reading

Lung Mechanics

Bhutani VK, Sivieri EM, Abbasi S, et al: Evaluation of neonatal pulmonary mechanics and energetics: a two factor least mean square analysis. *Pediatr Pulmonol* 1988;4:150-158.

Bryan AC, England SJ: Maintenance of an elevated FRC in the newborn: paradox of REM sleep. *Am Rev Respir Dis* 1984;129:209.

Cook CD, Sutherland JM, Segal S, et al: Studies of respiratory physiology in the newborn infant. III. Measurements of mechanics of respiration. *J Clin Invest* 1957;36:440.

Gerhardt T, Bancalari E: Chestwall compliance in full-term and premature infants. *Acta Paediatr Scand* 1980;69:359.

Lesouef PN, England SJ, Bryan AC: Passive respiratory mechanics in newborns and children. *Am Rev Respir Dis* 1984;129:552.

McCann EM, Goldman SL, Brady JP: Pulmonary function in the sick newborn infant. *Pediatr Res* 1987;21:313.

McIlroy MB, Tierney DF, Nadel JA: A new method for measurement of compliance and resistance of lungs and thorax. *J Appl Physiol* 1963;18:424.

Nelson NM: Neonatal pulmonary function. *Pediatr Clin North Am* 1966;13:769.

Nunn JF: *Nunn's Applied Respiratory Physiology*, 4th ed. Oxford, Butterworth Heinemann, 1993.

Perez-Fontan JJ, Heldt GP, Gregory GA: Resistance and inertia of endotracheal tubes used in infants during periodic flow. *Crit Care Med* 1985;13:1052-1055.

Polgar G, Promadhat V: *Pulmonary Function Testing in Children: Techniques and Standards.* Philadelphia, WB Saunders Co, 1971.

Richardson P, Pace WR, Valdes E, et al: Time dependence of lung mechanics in preterm lambs. *Pediatr Res* 1992;31:276-279.

Oxygen Transport and Alveolar Ventilation

Comroe JH, Forster RE II, Dubois AB, et al: *The Lung: Clinical Physiology and Pulmonary Function Tests.* 2nd ed. Chicago, Year Book Medical Publishers Inc, 1962, p 27.

Cook CD, Cherry RB, O'Brien D, et al: Studies of respiratory physiology in the newborn infant. I. Observations on normal premature and full-term infants. *J Clin Invest* 1955;34:975.

Nelson NM: Respiration and circulation after birth. In: Smith CA, Nelson NM, eds. *The Physiology of the Newborn Infant.* Springfield, Charles C Thomas, 1976.

Slonim NB, Hamilton LH: *Respiratory Physiology.* 5th ed. St Louis, CV Mosby, 1987, p 52.

Ventilation-Perfusion Relationships

Corbet AJS, Ross JA, Beaudry PH, et al: Effect of positive-pressure breathing on $aADn_2$ in hyaline membrane disease. *J Appl Physiol* 1975;38:33-38.

Corbet AJS, Ross JA, Beaudry PH, et al: Ventilation-perfusion relationships as assessed by $aADn_2$ in hyaline membrane disease. *J Appl Physiol* 1974;36:74-81.

Farhi LE: Ventilation-perfusion relationship and its role in alveolar gas exchange. In: Caro CG, ed. *Advances in Respiratory Physiology.* Baltimore, Williams and Wilkins, 1966.

Hansen TN, Corbet AJS, Kenny JD, et al: Effects of oxygen and constant positive pressure breathing on $aADCO_2$ in hyaline membrane disease. *Pediatr Res* 1979;13:1167-1171.

Landers S, Hansen TN, Corbet AJS, et al: Optimal constant positive airway pressure assessed by $aADCO_2$ in hyaline membrane disease. *Pediatr Res* 1986;20:884-889.

Markello R, Winter P, Olszowka A: Assessment of ventilation-perfusion inequalities by arterial-aveolar nitrogen differences in intensive care patients. *Anesthesiology* 1972;37:4.

Nelson NM: Respiration and circulation after birth. In: Smith CA, Nelson NM, eds. The *Physiology of the Newborn Infant.* Springfield, Charles C Thomas, 1976.

Nunn JF: *Nunn's Applied Respiratory Physiology,* 4th ed. Oxford, Butterworth Heinemann, 1993.

Thibeault DW, Poblete E, Auld PAM: Alveolar-arterial oxygen difference in premature infants breathing 100 per cent oxygen. *J Pediatr* 1967;71:814-824.

West JB: *Ventilation Blood Flow and Gas Exchange.* London, Blackwell Scientific, 1970.

Lung and Heart Interaction

Fishman AP: Pulmonary circulation. In: Fishman AP, Fisher AB, Geiger SR, eds. *Handbook of Physiology.* I. Bethesda, American Physiological Society, 1986, p 93.

McGregor M: Pulsus paradoxus. *N Engl J Med* 1979;301:480.

Niemann JT, Rosborough J, Hausknect M, et al: Cough-CPR: Documentation of systemic perfusion in man and in an experimental model: a 'window' to the mechanism of blood flow in external CPR. *Crit Care Med* 1980;8:141.

Perlman J, Thach B: Respiratory origin of fluctuations in arterial blood pressure in premature infants with respiratory distress syndrome. *Pediatrics* 1988;81:399.

Surfactant

Avery ME, Mead J: Surface properties in relation to atelectasis and hyaline membrane disease. *Am J Dis Child* 1959;97:517.

Bangham AD, Morley CJ, Phillips MC: The physical properties of an effective lung surfactant. *Biochim Biophys Acta* 1979;573:552.

Clements JA, Tooley WH: Kinetics of surface active material in the fetal lung. In: Hodson WA, ed. *Development of the Lung.* New York, Marcel Dekker Inc, 1977.

Clements JA: Surface phenomena in relation to pulmonary function (Sixth Bowditch Lecture). *Physiologist* 1962;5:11.

Gluck L, Kulovich MV, Borer RC, et al: Diagnosis of the respiratory distress syndrome by amniocentesis. *Am J Obstet Gynecol* 1971;109:440.

Goerke J: Lung surfactant. *Biochim Biophys Acta* 1974;344:241.

Hallman M, Gluck L: Development of the fetal lung. *J Perinat Med* 1977;5:3.

Hawgood S: Surfactant: composition, structure, and metabolism. In: Crystal RG, West JB, Barnes PJ, eds. *The Lung.* New York, Raven Press Ltd, 1991, p 247.

King RJ: Pulmonary surface active material: basic concepts. In: Bloom RS, Sinclair JC, Warshaw JB, eds. *The Surfactant and the Neonatal Lung.* Evansville, Mead Johnson and Co, 1979.

Smith BT: Pulmonary surfactant during fetal development and neonatal adaption: hormonal control. In: Robertson B, VanGolde LMG, Batenburg JJ, eds. *Pulmonary Surfactant.* Amsterdam, Elsevier Press, 1984.

VanGolde LMG, Batenburg JJ, Robertson B: The pulmonary surfactant system: biochemical aspects and functional significance. *Physiol Rev* 1988;68:374.

Whitsett JA: Pulmonary surfactant and respiratory distress syndrome in the premature infant. In: Crystal RG, West JB, Barnes PJ, eds. *The Lung.* New York, Raven Press Ltd, 1991, p 1723.

Chapter 3

Approach to the Patient With Respiratory Disease

A s in other areas of medicine, a good history and a thorough physical examination are essential to making an accurate diagnosis and to rendering the most appropriate management. In particular, antenatal and perinatal conditions may affect the risk and severity of respiratory distress (Tables 1 and 2). A systematic and complete maternal history is essential to anticipate problems and optimize care to high-risk newborns. The following is a suggested list of items to include in a complete history.

History
Maternal History

- Health before this pregnancy (including during previous pregnancies)
- Prenatal care (including date of first visit, number of visits, weight gain, and laboratory and ultrasound studies)
- Family illnesses, including father's family
- Pregnancy-related illnesses (eg, diabetes, pregnancy-induced hypertension, sexually transmitted diseases, or infections)
- Maternal medications (including vitamins and iron) and substance abuse (eg, cigarettes, alcohol, or street drugs)
- Time and reason for maternal admission to the hospital
- Time of onset of labor
- Maternal evaluation and treatment since admission (eg, antibiotics, corticosteroids, tocolytics, or narcotics)

Table 1: Risk Factors Associated With Hyaline Membrane Disease

Increased risk	Decreased risk
Male sex	Female sex
White race	Black race
L/S ratio <2.0 in prematures	L/S ratio >2.0
Previously affected sibling	Maternal toxemia
Maternal diabetes (class A, B, or C)	Maternal diabetes (class D, F, or R)
Maternal hypotension	Maternal drug abuse
C-section without labor	Maternal antenatal corticosteroids
Third-trimester hemorrhage	Chronic abruption
Second twin	Prolonged rupture of membranes
Hydrops fetalis	Intrauterine growth retardation
Fetal depression	

- Fetal status, including time of rupture of membranes, description of amniotic fluid (clear, foul smelling, or meconium stained), maternal bleeding (timing and amount), and evidence of fetal distress
- Method of delivery (cesarean [C-section] or vaginal)
- Gestational age at delivery and (determination) method

History of the Infant
- Condition at delivery (resuscitation, Apgar score, and Silverman score)
- Admission vital signs
- Observations, evaluations, and treatment during the period of neonatal transition and before consultation

By Charleta Guillory, MD, and Gerardo Cabrera-Meza, MD

Table 2: Risk Factors Associated With Other Diseases

Associated With Other Lung Diseases

Congenital pneumonia	Male sex
	Maternal fever
	Chorioamnionitis
	Preterm labor
	Prolonged labor
	Maternal colonization with group B streptococci
	Tracheoesophageal fistula
Meconium aspiration syndrome	Meconium-stained amniotic fluid
	Fetal depression
	Postmaturity
Transient tachypnea of the newborn	Term infants
	Delivery by C-section
	Rapid labor
	Perinatal depression

Physical Examination

Examination of the respiratory system of the newborn includes inspection, palpation, and auscultation.

Inspection

Nutrition. A wasted appearance suggests placental insufficiency and an infant at risk for persistent pulmonary hypertension, while a large-for-gestational-age infant may be an infant of a diabetic mother and be at risk for hyaline membrane disease (HMD).

Skin. The presence and distribution of cyanosis should be determined by examination while the infant is quiet and

Associated With Other Lung Diseases

Persistent pulmonary Meconium aspiration
  hypertension of   syndrome
  the newborn   Perinatal depression
              Pneumonia
              Polycythemia
              Congenital diaphragmatic hernia
              Maternal aspirin therapy
              Hyaline membrane disease
              Cold stress

Associated With Congenital Anomalies

Polyhydramnios   Diaphragmatic hernia
              Tracheoesophageal fistula

Oligohydramnios   Pulmonary hypoplasia
              Prolonged rupture of membranes
              Renal agenesis

in a well-lighted area. Cyanosis of only the hands and feet (acrocyanosis) is a normal finding during the first days after birth. Central cyanosis (cyanosis of the tongue, mucous membranes, and skin) is abnormal in the noncrying infant after the first few minutes of age; it occurs when the concentration of deoxygenated hemoglobin exceeds 3 g/dL and strongly suggests hypoxemia. The presence of pallor suggests shock, cutaneous vasoconstriction, obstruction of cardiac output (eg, aortic stenosis), or anemia. Plethora, meconium staining, or exanthems suggest polycythemia, meconium aspiration syndrome, or pneumonia, respectively, as the etiology of respiratory distress.

Table 3: Causes of Changes in Chest Volume

Bilateral change in chest volume

Increased chest volume	*Decreased chest volume*
Transient tachypnea	Hyaline membrane disease
Meconium aspiration pneumonia	Pulmonary hypoplasia
Persistent pulmonary hypertension of the newborn	Chest wall restriction
Cystic lung diseases	

Nose. The alae nasae is the first muscle activated during inspiration. Nasal flaring represents an attempt to decrease airway resistance and is a sign of air hunger.

Chest: Size, shape, and symmetry. A barrel-shaped chest suggests increased lung volume, while a bell-shaped chest may be seen with reduced lung volume. Chest wall asymmetry results from volume differences between the two sides of the thoracic cavity. While the side that *appears* to bulge may be either normal or abnormal (Table 3), the normal side of the chest will usually rise and fall the most with spontaneous respirations.

Retractions. The chest wall of the infant, especially the extremely low-birth-weight infant ($\leq$1,000 g), is extremely compliant. With spontaneous breathing, the pleural pressure (Ppl) decreases during inspiration. Infants with parenchymal disease, such as HMD or transient tachypnea of the newborn (TTN), must produce a more negative Ppl than normal. Consequently, the highly compliant chest wall may cave inward as a result of these more negative pressures. Moderate decreases in Ppl result in intercostal and xiphoid retractions, while marked decreases result in collapse of the entire upper

Unilateral increase in chest volume

Pathology on the low-volume side	*Pathology on the high-volume side*
Atelectasis	Pneumothorax
Unilateral pulmonary hypoplasia	Unilateral interstitial emphysema
	Cystic lung disease
	Diaphragmatic hernia
	Chylothorax

chest. This collapse, coupled with the outward displacement of the abdominal contents by the descending diaphragm, results in the characteristic see-saw breathing pattern of severe respiratory distress. Retractions are an external estimate of Ppl and are predictive of the severity of respiratory distress. While airway obstruction can cause retractions, the most common cause is reduced lung compliance, usually from HMD.

Respiratory rate. The respiratory rate should be counted for 1 full minute. Tachypnea, a resting rate >60 breaths/min, is the most sensitive single sign of respiratory distress.

Respiratory pattern. Many normal premature (and some term) infants exhibit periodic breathing, which consists of bursts of respirations followed by cessation of respiratory efforts (apnea) lasting 5 to 10 seconds (see *Control of Breathing*, Chapter 9.)

Heart. The point of maximum impact (PMI) of the heart is often visible. The PMI will shift away from a space-occupying lesion or toward an area of volume loss.

Abdomen. A scaphoid, empty abdomen is a classic presentation for the infant with congenital diaphragmatic hernia or for the asphyxiated infant who has passed meconium in utero. A distended abdomen may signal a tracheoesophageal fistula, particularly in infants receiving positive pressure ventilation.

A shift of the umbilicus toward one side during inspiration, the 'belly dancer's sign,' suggests a paralyzed diaphragm on the side of the shift. As the functioning diaphragmatic leaf descends, the other leaf is pulled up by the falling Ppl into the chest, pulling the abdominal contents and umbilicus with it.

Palpation

Overinflated lungs can displace the liver and spleen from beneath the rib margins and make them more easily detected by abdominal palpation. An enlarged, tense abdomen or a large abdominal mass can compromise the diaphragm's descent.

Auscultation

Grunting. Infants with respiratory distress often grunt by opposing their vocal cords at the end of expiration. The grunt produces a positive end expiratory pressure that splints small airways open and improves the distribution of ventilation. The louder the grunt, the more severe the respiratory distress.

Stridor. Stridor suggests large airway obstruction. With intrathoracic airway obstruction, expiration tends to narrow the airway, making the expiratory component of stridor worse. Conversely, with extrathoracic airway obstruction, *inspiratory* stridor is usually worse.

Breath sounds. Breath sounds can be evaluated for strength, duration, and symmetry as well as for rales, rhonchi, or wheezes. Breath sounds may be symmetrically decreased in diseases with poor air entry, such as HMD or pulmonary hypoplasia. The duration of audible, expiratory breath sounds provides information about the expiratory time constant and expiratory airway resistance. If expiration visibly ceases after one to two time constants, the observed expiratory time may be used to estimate the time constant for expiration and expiratory resistance (see *Lung*

Table 4: The Silverman Score			
Sign	0	1	2
Upper Chest	Synchronized with lower chest	Lag on inspiration	See-saw
Lower chest retractions	None	Just visible	Marked
Xiphoid retraction	None	Just visible	Marked
Nasal flaring	None	Minimal	Marked
Expiratory grunt	None	Heard only with stethoscope	Audible with naked ear

Mechanics, Chapter 2). In asymmetric lung diseases, breath sounds are usually loudest over the normal side of the chest (Table 3).

While rales and rhonchi are nonspecific in the infant with respiratory distress, wheezing, which is more common in older infants with bronchopulmonary dysplasia or pneumonia, usually indicates significant airway obstruction.

Silverman Score

This scoring system (Table 4) may be used to quantitate the severity of respiratory distress. An infant with mild respiratory distress scores 2 to 4, while one with severe distress scores 8 to 10.

Transillumination

Transillumination can be valuable for detecting asymmetries of the chest. An increase in transillumination on one side suggests a pneumothorax in an acutely deteriorating infant (see *Air Block* section, Chapter 5).

By Charleta Guillory, MD, and Gerardo Carbrera-Meza, MD

X-ray Patterns in Neonatal Lung Disease: Phases of Chest X-ray

The clinical presentation of many respiratory and nonrespiratory diseases may appear similar; accurately diagnosing the etiology is difficult without chest radiographs. Careful, methodic evaluation of the radiograph is essential. Important clues, or unsuspected complications, can be overlooked if the clinician focuses on only a portion of the chest radiograph. The single best view to obtain is the anteroposterior view. A cross-table lateral or lateral decubitus view can be helpful in the diagnosis of a pneumothorax or for confirmation of chest tube position.

Evaluation
Proper Technique and Positioning

Check for proper penetration and symmetry and for proper positioning of the x-ray tube over the baby. Penetration may be evaluated by comparing the densities of the vertebral bodies and the interspace between them. Rotation of the infant may be manifested by asymmetric clavicles, spine, and the anterior projection of the ribs. Improper angling of the x-ray tube nonperpendicular to the plane of the baby can produce bizarre rib patterns: with lordotic positioning, the x-ray tube is aimed toward the head, and the subsequent radiograph will display horizontal ribs and a tetralogy-like cardiac silhouette. If the tube is aimed toward the feet, the ribs can take on a bizarre, fanlike appearance.

Noncardiopulmonary Features

Common normal findings and variations should be noted (Table 5).

Systematically evaluate the bones, soft tissues, and visible portions of the abdomen before concentrating on the heart and lungs. With each radiograph, check for catheter and tube position because these may not remain constant during the neonatal intensive care unit course. Skin folds, the most com-

Table 5: Common Chest Radiograph Findings and Variations

Normal findings	Normal variations
Uniform lung fields	Pleural fissures
Hilar markings less prominent than in child	Tracheal buckling and indentations
Eighth-ninth rib expansion	Mediastinal lines
Right-sided deviation of trachea	Pseudohyperlucent lung
Air bronchograms	Intercostal or apical herniation
Cardiac silhouette <60% of chest	Suprasternal fossa

mon artifact, result from the folding of redundant skin. They may be mistaken for pneumothoraces, especially if they lie parallel to the chest wall and do not cross outside the thorax. This may be differentiated from a pneumothorax by the presence of vascular markings and the absence of the hyperlucent field lateral to the edge of the collapsed lung seen in a pneumothorax. Radiographs taken through the walls of an incubator may show the hole in the incubator as a pseudocyst. Of course, this marking will be entirely symmetric and smooth-edged and will not be found in previous or subsequent radiographs. In infants with respiratory distress and suprasternal retractions, the suprasternal fossa can appear as a radiolucency, which may be difficult to distinguish from the proximal esophageal pouch of an infant with esophageal atresia.

Airway Features

The trachea and major bronchi are well distended with deep inspiration or positive pressure ventilation. Because of the increased flexibility of the neonate's trachea, compared

Table 6: Differential Diagnoses of Abnormal Radiograph Patterns

Clear or dark lungs with respiratory distress	Metabolic causes Central nervous system injury Cardiac disease Persistent pulmonary hypertension Hypoplastic lungs
Grainy lungs	Hyaline membrane disease Poorly ventilated lungs Transient tachypnea of the newborn Pneumonia Partial anomalous pulmonary venous return with obstruction
Hazy or patchy lungs	Pulmonary hemorrhagic edema Pneumonia (usually viral) Chronic pulmonary insufficiency of the premature Early bronchopulmonary dysplasia, Northway stage II
Increased vascular markings	Transient tachypnea of the newborn Meconium aspiration Congenital heart disease with congestive heart failure Pulmonary edema Pulmonary lymphangiectasia Viral pneumonitis

with the older child, normal variations in the trachea are common and include narrowing of the trachea (which may appear striking) or anterior buckling of the airway (which may mimic the presence of a retropharyngeal mass). The trachea will usually deviate toward the right. Air bronchograms may

Reticulonodular lungs	Pneumonia
	Meconium aspiration
	Wilson-Mikity syndrome
	Early bronchopulmonary dysplasia
Bubbly lungs	
Small bubbles	HMD
	Pulmonary interstitial emphysema
	Bronchopulmonary dysplasia, early
Large bubbles	Bronchopulmonary dysplasia, late
	Pneumatoceles with pneumonia
	Cystic adenomatoid malformation
	Congenital lobar emphysema
	Bronchogenic cysts
	Congenital diaphragmatic hernia
Opaque lungs	Expiratory phase of HMD
	Primary atelectasis
	Pulmonary agenesis
	Massive pulmonary hemorrhagic edema—rare
	Bilateral chylothorax or hydrothorax—rare
	Weak, depressed infant with poor respiratory effort

be present, especially behind the cardiac silhouette. While airway abnormalities may be visible on plain radiographs, magnetic resonance imaging, computed tomography, or bronchography are usually required for definitive radiographic diagnosis.

Gastrointestinal Features

Air is commonly seen within the esophagus; however, persistent or prominent esophageal air collections may be seen with an H-type tracheoesophageal fistula or esophageal reflux. In infants with esophageal atresia, an enlarged, air-filled proximal pouch will usually be found.

Cardiopulmonary Features

The clinician should evaluate the heart and lungs for overall lung expansion and symmetry, for degree of pulmonary vascularity, for general parenchymal pattern (eg, clear, hazy, streaky, nodular, or cystic), and for the presence of abnormal masses or extraparenchymal collections of air. Normal pulmonary parenchyma will have symmetric, uniform, radiolucent-appearing fields with perihilar markings increasingly present over the medial portion of the lung field. Over the lateral lung fields, pulmonary vasculature usually will be barely noticeable. Evaluating for overall lung expansion is difficult. With a good inspiration, the normal lung will be expanded to the level of the posterior aspect of the eighth to ninth ribs. The posterior aspect of the ribs will project downward.

Normal variations of the lungs are commonly noted. Visualization of the interlobar fissures, especially the right minor fissure, is reported in as many as 70% of cases. The right, posterior reflection of the pleura is sometimes visualized as a mediastinal line. This is best seen on overpenetrated radiographs. Rotation of the chest may result in a pseudohyperlucent hemithorax.

Abnormalities in expansion and parenchymal patterns are very helpful in limiting the differential diagnosis under consideration (Table 6). In particular, it is helpful to evaluate the lungs for general radiodensity (dark or hazy), for variations in density (diffuse patchy infiltrates, increased density appearing to be composed of grainlike particles, or bubbly areas of hyperlucency), and for distribution of abnormalities (perihilar, peripheral, or lobar).

When evaluating streaky lungs with radiating, linear densities, differentiate air bronchograms (dark lines projected on a gray background, especially common over the cardiac silhouette, and generally seen only in the perihilar area) from exaggerated vasculature (light lines on a gray background, often with a lacy distribution, and extending farther to the periphery). Air bronchograms, normal if involving only the trachea and major bronchi, are common with primary parenchymal disease. Exaggerated vasculature is often seen secondary to engorged lymphatic vessels from transient tachypnea of the newborn (TTN) or pulmonary edema.

By Timothy R. Cooper, MD

Pulmonary Function Testing

In the past, measurements of compliance, resistance, and lung volumes were confined to the research laboratory. However, several commercial systems for measuring lung function have recently become available and have proven clinically useful. Clinical interpretation of the results of these tests, however, requires an understanding of their physiologic basis.

Measurements of Compliance and Resistance

Static compliance. In infants, *static compliance* is measured by instilling a known volume of gas into the lung through a face mask or endotracheal tube and measuring the change in distending pressure (Table 7):

$$\text{Compliance} = \Delta \text{ volume} / \Delta \text{ pressure}$$

Alveolar pressure cannot be measured directly but is equal to airway pressure when there is no gas flow in or out of the lung (see *Lung Mechanics*, Chapter 2). For measurements of *static lung compliance*, alveolar pressure is measured by occluding the airway until gas flow ceases and then measuring airway pressure with a pressure transducer connected to the upper airway via a face mask or endotracheal tube. This occlusion may last several seconds. Pleural pressure is measured using a pressure transducer connected to a balloon cath-

Table 7: Distending Pressures for Measurements of Compliance

Compliance	Distending Pressure	Simplified Distending Pressure *
Lung	Alveolar - Pleural pressure	Airway - Pleural pressure
Chest wall	Pleural - Atmospheric pressure	Pleural pressure
Respiratory system	Alveolar - Atmospheric pressure	Airway pressure*

* The distending pressures can be simplified using the following assumptions:

  Airway pressure equals alveolar pressure when there is no gas flow in or out of the lung.

  Atmospheric pressure, the reference pressure, equals zero.

eter placed in the distal esophagus. Measurements of distending pressure are repeated at multiple inflation volumes and pressure-volume curves are constructed (Chapter 2, Figures 1, 3). Compliance is calculated from the slope of the curve. Since this technique is difficult to perform in the spontaneously breathing infant, other more clinically useful measurements of compliance have been developed.

Passive exhalation. The passive exhalation (Figure 1) technique measures compliance and resistance of the *respiratory system*. For this measurement, the infant's airway is occluded at the end of either a spontaneous or positive pressure breath and airway pressure is measured to estimate alveolar pressure. Airway pressure is measured using a pres-

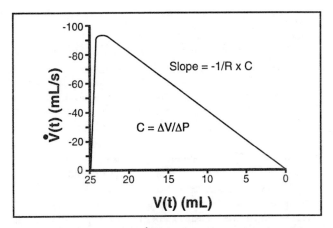

Figure 1: Expiratory flow ($\dot{V}[t]$) is plotted as a function of lung volume above functional residual capacity, V(t). During expiration, the lung volume above functional residual capacity decreases over time. The lung has a resistance = 0.05 cm H_2O/mL/s and compliance = 5 mL/cm H_2O. Gas flow out of the lung is negative by convention. The slope of the line is the negative reciprocal of the time constant (R x C). Compliance can be calculated from measurements of exhaled volume (ΔV) and airway pressure measured immediately before exhalation (ΔP). (Adapted from Hansen TN, Corbet AJ. In: Taeusch HW, et al, eds. *Schaffer and Avery's Diseases of the Newborn*. 5th ed. Philadelphia, WB Saunders, 1991.)

sure transducer connected to the upper airway via a face mask or endotracheal tube. The airway is then opened and the lungs are allowed to passively deflate, while exhaled gas flow rate is measured using a pneumotachometer in line with the face mask or endotracheal tube. The pneumotachometer has a fixed internal resistance; as gas flows out of the infant's lung across this resistance, a pressure differential is created. The magnitude of this pressure differential is directly proportional to the rate of flow. These *measurements of flow* can be electronically integrated to give *measurements of volume* of gas entering and leaving the lung.

During a passive exhalation, proximal airway pressure equals atmospheric pressure, which equals zero. Therefore, the equation of motion (see *Lung Mechanics*, Chapter 2) simplifies to $V(t)/C + \dot{V}(t) \times R = 0$. Rearranging this equation gives $\dot{V}(t) = (-1/R \times C) \times V(t)$ where $\dot{V}(t)$ is the rate of gas flow out of the lung at time t. $V(t)$ is the lung volume at time t. As expected from Figure 1, this is the equation of a straight line, $y = mx + b$, where y is $\dot{V}(t)$, x is $V(t)$, m is the slope, $-1/R \times C$, and the intercept, b, is zero. *Compliance* of the respiratory system is calculated by dividing the exhaled volume by the airway pressure measured at the end of the airway occlusion. Since the airway occlusion during this maneuver may not be sufficiently long to ensure cessation of gas flow and a true measurement of alveolar pressure, this is a measurement of *quasistatic lung compliance*. The *respiratory time constant* is calculated from the slope of the line $(-1/R \times C)$, and *respiratory system resistance* is calculated by dividing the time constant by the compliance.

Dynamic measurements of resistance and compliance. Compliance and resistance can also be calculated from measurements of pressure, inspiratory and expiratory flow, and volume (Figure 2).

In the spontaneously breathing infant (Figure 2), *lung compliance* can be calculated by dividing the volume of gas entering the lung during a tidal breath by the change in distending pressure. There is no gas flow in and out of the lung at end inspiration and end expiration, so at these points alveolar pressure equals airway pressure, which equals zero. Therefore, the change in distending pressure is equal to the change in pleural pressure (Table 7 and Figure 2).

In patients undergoing positive-pressure ventilation, the distending pressure for the *lung* is alveolar pressure minus pleural pressure, while distending pressure for the *respiratory system* is alveolar pressure minus atmospheric pressure. Again, alveolar pressure is assumed to be equal to airway pressure at points of no gas flow (end inspiration and end

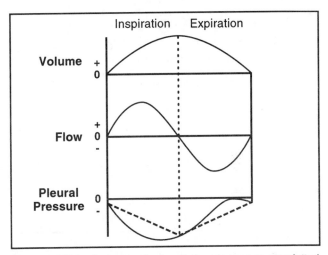

Figure 2: Tidal volume, gas flow, and pleural pressure are plotted for a spontaneous inspiration and expiration. During inspiration, the thorax expands, pleural pressure decreases (becomes more negative), the lung expands, and alveolar pressure decreases. Gas flows from the atmosphere through the airways into the alveoli and the volume of gas in the lungs increases. Gas flow into the lungs is positive by convention. Gas continues to flow until alveolar pressure equals atmospheric pressure, at which point gas flow, hence inspiration, ceases. During expiration, the thorax relaxes, pleural pressure increases, alveolar pressure increases, gas flows from the lung into the atmosphere, and lung volume decreases. Gas flow out of the lung is negative by convention. Gas continues to flow out of the lung until alveolar pressure equals atmospheric pressure, at which point gas flow, hence expiration, ceases. The dashed line shows the pleural pressure required to overcome elastic forces alone.

expiration). Thus, distending pressure for the lung is airway pressure minus intrapleural pressure, and distending pressure for the respiratory system is airway pressure.

For all of these measurements, pressures, gas flows, and volumes are measured as described in the two previous sec-

Table 8: Distribution of Alveolar Volumes and Pressures With Increasing Respiratory Rate

RR/ min	IT sec	Volume A mL	Alveolar Pressure A cm H_2O
20	1.5	20	20
30	1.0	20	20
60	0.5	20	20
75	0.4	20	20

Volumes are determined from graphs in Figure 3.

tions. Since all measurements of distending pressure are made while the infant is breathing, the period of no gas flow at end inspiration and end expiration is quite brief. Therefore, these measurements are referred to as measurements of *dynamic compliance*.

Resistance is calculated by picking points of equal inspiratory and expiratory volume on a tracing similar to Figure 2 and measuring gas flow and pleural pressure at these points. Since the elastic components of driving pressure at points of equal lung volume are identical, they cancel out and leave resistance as the only force opposing gas movement. *Mean lung resistance* is equal to the driving pressure at the inspiratory point minus the driving pressure at the expiratory point divided by the sum of the inspiratory and expiratory flow rates.

More recently, investigators have calculated airway resistance and compliance by measuring distending pressure, gas flow, and volume continuously and then fitting these values to the equation of motion using multiple linear regression techniques to derive the constants 1/C and R. Obviously, these techniques measure *dynamic compliance*.

Volume B mL	Alveolar Pressure B cm H_2O	Total Volume mL	Total Compliance mL/cm H_2O
20	20	40	2.0
18	18	38	1.9
14	14	34	1.7
12	12	32	1.6

Specific lung compliance. Measured lung compliance is markedly affected by size. For example, a 3-kg infant with a lung compliance of 2 mL/cm H_2O requires a 10 cm H_2O distending pressure to deliver a tidal volume of 20 mL. Conversely, the same 10 cm H_2O distending pressure in an adult delivers a tidal volume of 500 mL and results in a lung compliance of 50 mL/cm H_2O. In fact, the elastic properties of the adult and newborn lung are almost equal, but the adult lung is much larger. To correct for lung size, the *specific compliance* is calculated by dividing measured compliance by the functional residual capacity (90 mL for a 3-kg infant and 2,000 mL for an adult). With this correction, the infant and adult both have compliances of about 25 mL/cm H_2O/L lung volume.

Frequency dependence of lung compliance. Measurements of dynamic lung compliance rely on the assumption that at end inspiration and expiration, gas flow in the lung ceases and alveolar pressure equals airway pressure. In the presence of ventilation inhomogeneities, this assumption is not true (Figure 3). In Figure 3, the lung is composed of two ventilatory compartments—one well ventilated (A) and the other poorly ventilated (B).

This lung is ventilated with an airway pressure of 20 cm H_2O, a fixed inspiratory to expiratory time ratio of 1:1, and progressively greater respiratory rates (RR). As RR increases, inspiratory time (IT) decreases (Table 8). The volume of gas entering the well-ventilated lung compartment (A) is not affected by decreasing IT. However, as IT decreases, the volume of gas entering the poorly ventilated compartment (B) decreases, decreasing the total volume of gas entering the lung. In this example, dynamic compliance is calculated by dividing the total volume of gas in the lung at end inspiration by the peak airway pressure of 20 cm H_2O. Dynamic compliance decreases with increasing RR (decreasing IT). The decrease in dynamic compliance measured with increasing respiratory rates is termed *frequency dependence of lung compliance.*

Alveolar pressure can be calculated for each compartment by dividing the volume of gas in the compartment by its compliance. In the well-ventilated compartment (A), alveolar pressure is equal to airway pressure, but in the poorly ventilated compartment (B), alveolar pressure equals airway pressure only at the slowest RR chosen.

Static compliance could have been measured at an RR of 60 breaths/min by occluding the airway at end inspiration for 2 to 3 seconds. During this occlusion, gas would actually flow from the well-ventilated compartment (A) along the alveolar pressure gradient into compartment (B) until the volumes in each compartment were equal at 17 mL. This redistribution of gas within the lung is called *pendelluft.* After this redistribution, the alveolar pressures in A and B would be equal, and the measured airway pressure would be 17 cm H_2O. Static lung compliance would then be calculated by dividing total lung volume (C) by the airway pressure (34 mL/17 cm H_2O = 2 mL/cm H_2O). This static lung compliance differs from the dynamic lung compliance because of pendelluft.

The phenomenon of frequency dependence of compliance often results in measurements of dynamic lung compliance

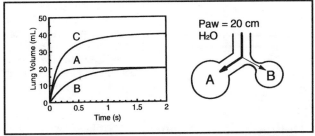

Figure 3: The figure on the right depicts a two-compartment lung (see table). The lung is being ventilated with a peak airway pressure of 20 cm H_2O. The table describes the functional characteristics of each lung compartment. The figure graphically represents the volume-time relationships of these compartments.

Compartment	Compliance (mL/cm H_2O)	Resistance (cm H_2O/mL/s)	Time Constant (s)	Vmax (mL)
A	1.0	0.10	0.10	20
B	1.0	0.40	0.40	20

The two lung compartments have equal lung compliances. Compartment B has a much higher airway resistance than compartment A, and the time constant for compartment B is four times that of compartment A. Consequently, the rate of gas flow into compartment B is much less than for compartment A. Since lung compliance and airway pressure are the same for both compartments, both will eventually inflate to the same maximum lung volume (Vmax); Vmax = compliance x peak airway pressure. However, it will take four times as long for compartment B to reach Vmax as it does for compartment A. The total amount of gas in the lung at any time is equal to the sum of the volumes of gas in each compartment. Volume in C = Volume in A + Volume in B.

that are less than measurements of static lung compliance. In fact, measurements of dynamic lung compliance are often more affected by airway dysfunction than they are by changes in lung elasticity.

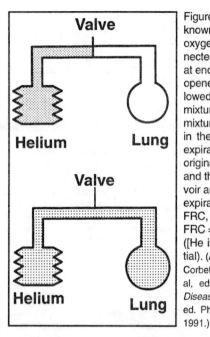

Figure 4: A reservoir with a known amount of helium in oxygen (He initial) is connected to the infant's airway; at end expiration the valve is opened and the infant is allowed to breathe the gas mixture. The helium oxygen mixture is diluted by the gas in the infant's lungs at end expiration (He final). If the original helium concentration and the volume of the reservoir are both known, the end expiratory lung volume, or FRC, is given by:
FRC = Reservoir volume x ([He initial - He final]/He initial). (Adapted from Hansen TN, Corbet AJ. In: Taeusch HW, et al, eds. *Schaffer and Avery's Diseases of the Newborn*. 5th ed. Philadelphia, WB Saunders, 1991.)

Measurements of Functional Residual Capacity

Functional residual capacity (FRC) can be measured directly using an inert gas dilution technique or as thoracic gas volume using a plethysmograph. The most common clinical method for measurement of FRC is helium dilution (Figure 4).

By W. Scott Jarriel, MD, and Thomas N. Hansen, MD

Differentiation of Heart and Lung Disease

Differentiating between heart and lung disease in a cyanotic newborn is a frequent and sometimes difficult problem that requires systematic evaluation.

Cyanosis

The clinician must determine if cyanosis is pathologic or physiologic.

Table 9: Causes of Hypoxemia	
Cause of Hypoxemia	**Associated Disorders**
Hypoventilation	Loss of respiratory drive Mechanical interference with lung inflation
Ventilation/perfusion mismatch	Parenchymal lung disease
Right-to-left shunt	Congenital heart disease Persistent pulmonary hypertension
Methemoglobinemia	Abnormal hemoglobin Nitrate toxicity

Central cyanosis will present as a blue discoloration of tongue, mucous membranes, extremities, and skin. The appearance of cyanosis depends on the absolute concentration of reduced hemoglobin in the blood, not the ratio of reduced to oxygenated hemoglobin. Three grams or more of reduced hemoglobin are required to produce visible cyanosis. Central cyanosis is abnormal in the quiet newborn after 20 minutes of age. However, it may be seen in normal infants with crying for several days after birth secondary to right-to-left shunting through the foramen ovale.

Peripheral cyanosis (acrocyanosis), which is blue discoloration of the skin of the extremities, is common in normal newborns for days to weeks. Peripheral cyanosis with cold extremities in a warm environment could suggest vasoconstriction in a septic infant or an infant in heart failure.

Causes of Hypoxemia

If central cyanosis is present on physical examination, the infant's oxygenation should be assessed by pulse oximetry, measurement of transcutaneous Po_2, or measurement of oxygen tension in a sample of arterial blood. In most instances, central cyanosis will be accompanied by arterial hypoxemia. The exception to this occurs with methemoglobinemia. Potential causes of hypoxemia/cyanosis are listed in Table 9.

Diagnostic Approach

History. Infants with hypoxemia secondary to hypoventilation are usually premature or are depressed at birth secondary to maternal medications or difficult delivery. Infants with parenchymal lung disease have a history compatible with the underlying disorder, ie, prematurity, meconium staining, etc. Infants with persistent pulmonary hypertension (PPHN) often have a history of meconium staining, perinatal asphyxia, or risk factors for sepsis/pneumonia. Interestingly, infants with cyanotic congenital heart disease often present in the newborn nursery after an uncomplicated labor and delivery. Finally, infants with methemoglobinemia may have a history of exposure to nitrates.

Physical Examination

Respiratory pattern. Infants with central hypoventilation will have shallow respirations and may have periodic breathing with apneic pauses. Chest wall abnormalities that interfere with lung expansion should be obvious. Infants with parenchymal lung disease will have tachypnea, grunting, and signs of altered lung compliance such as chest wall retractions and see-saw respirations. Infants with cyanotic congenital heart disease will usually present without tachypnea or the appearance of respiratory distress. Infants with PPHN and little parenchymal lung involvement may have a similar presentation.

Auscultation. Breath sounds are often decreased in infants with hypoventilation or parenchymal lung disease. Infants in the latter category may also have rales. The value of asymmetric breath sounds is covered in detail in the section on physical examination at the beginning of this chapter. The presence or absence of a murmur may help alert the physician to the possibility of congenital heart disease.

Table 10: Arterial Blood Gas Tensions in Infants with Hypoxemia

Cause of Hypoxemia	Typical Arterial Blood Gas Findings
Hypoventilation	Increased $Paco_2$
	Supplemental O_2 increases Pao_2
Ventilation/perfusion mismatch	$Paco_2$ normal to decreased
	Breathing 100% O_2 increases Pao_2
	Increased MAP increases Pao_2
Right-to-left shunt	$Paco_2$ normal to decreased
	Breathing 100% O_2 does not increase Pao_2
	Increased MAP does not increase Pao_2
	For infants with PPHN, hyperventilation and increased arterial pH may increase Pao_2
Methemoglobinemia	Pao_2 normal
	O_2 saturation decreased
	Arterial blood remains brown upon direct exposure to O_2*

* A spot of blood placed on a piece of paper that remains chocolate brown should raise suspicions of methemoglobinemia.

Laboratory

General. A hematocrit should be obtained to rule out polycythemia. A serum glucose level should be obtained to determine the presence of hypoglycemia, which may be primary but more often accompanies either cyanotic congenital heart disease or parenchymal lung disease.

Arterial blood gases. Arterial blood gas tensions are often very helpful in discerning the cause of hypoxemia (Table 10). The measurements may be obtained using one of the noninvasive methods discussed in Chapter 10, or by obtaining samples of arterial blood.

Chest radiograph. The chest radiograph is sometimes useful in distinguishing congenital heart disease from primary parenchymal lung disease. A large heart with clear lung fields suggests congenital heart disease but could also accompany PPHN. On the other hand, while primary lung disease will usually have a normal size heart and abnormal lung fields, certain types of congenital heart disease, notably transposition of the great vessels and anomalous pulmonary venous return, may present with pulmonary edema.

Other tests. If congenital heart disease cannot be definitely ruled out using the tests outlined above, an ECG, echocardiogram, and cardiology consultation should be obtained. If there is still not a definitive diagnosis, then cardiac catheterization should be performed.

By Alica A. Moïse, MD, and Alfred L. Gest, MD

Suggested Reading
History and Physical Examination

Ballard JL, et al: A simplified assessment of gestational age. *Pediatr Res* 1977;11:374.

Bates B: *A Guide to Physical Diagnosis and History Taking.* 4th ed. Philadelphia, JB Lippincott, 1987.

Graham J: *Smith's Recognizable Patterns of Human Deformation.* Philadelphia, WB Saunders Co, 1988.

Oski F, DeAngelis C, Feigin R, et al: *Principles and Practice of Pediatrics.* Philadelphia, JB Lippincott, 1990.

Scanlon J: *A System of Newborn Physical Exam.* Baltimore, University Park Press, 1979.

Heart and Lung Interaction

Adams JM: Neonatology. In: Garson A, Bricker JT, McNamara DG, eds. *The Science and Practice of Pediatric Cardiology*. Philadelphia, Lea & Febiger, pp 2477-2490, 1990.

Bancalari E, Jesse MJ, Gelband H, et al: Lung mechanics in congenital heart disease with increased and decreased pulmonary blood flow. *J Pediatr* 1977;90:192.

Dudell GG, Gersony WM: Patent ductus arteriosus in neonates with severe respiratory distress. *J Pediatr* 1984;104:915.

Fisher DJ: Oxygenation and metabolism in the developing heart. *Semin Perinatol* 1984;8:217.

Goldman HI, Maralit A, Sun S, et al: Neonatal cyanosis and arterial oxygen saturations. *J Pediatr* 1973;82:319-324.

Johnson GL: Clinical examination. In: Long WA, ed. *Fetal & Neonatal Cardiology*. Philadelphia, WB Saunders Co, pp 223-235, 1990.

Chest Radiographs

Avery ME, Gatewood OB, Brumley G: Transient tachypnea of the newborn: possible delayed resorption of fluid at birth. *Am J Dis Child* 1966; 11:380.

Ellis K, Nadelhaft J: Roentgenographic findings in hyaline membrane disease in infants weighing 2,000 grams and over. *Am J Roentgenol Radium Ther Nucl Med* 1957;78:444.

Emery JL: Interstitial emphysema, pneumothorax, and "air-block" in the newborn. *Lancet* 1956;1:405.

Loher E, Giedion A: Radiological aspects of massive hemorrhage in the newborn: report of three surviving cases. *Ann Radiol* 1971;14:147.

Mikity VG, Hodgman JE, Tatter D: The radiologic findings in delayed pulmonary maturation in premature infants. In: Kaufman HJ, ed. *Pediatric Radiology*. Chicago, Year Book, p 149, 1967.

Northway WH Jr, Rosan RC: The radiographic features of pulmonary oxygen toxicity in the newborn: bronchopulmonary dysplasia. *Radiology* 1968;91:49.

Swischuk LE: Bubbles in hyaline membrane disease (differentiation of three types). *Radiology* 1977;122:417.

Swischuck LE: Radiology of pulmonary insufficiency. In: Thibeault DW, Gregory GA, eds. *Neonatal Pulmonary Care*. 2nd ed. Appleton-Century-Crofts, 1986, pp 235-280.

Thibeault DW, Grossman H, Hagstrom JWC, et al: Radiologic findings in the lungs of premature infants. *J Pediatr* 1969;74:1.

Vollman JH, Smith WL, Ballard ET, et al: Early onset group B streptococcal disease: clinical, roentgenographic and pathologic features. *J Pediatr* 1976;89:199.

Wesenberg RL, Graven SN, McCabe EB: Radiological findings in wet-lung disease. *Radiology* 1971;98:69.

Wesenberg RL, Wax RE, Zachman RD: Varying roentgenographic patterns of patent ductus arteriosus in the newborn. *Am J Roentgenol Radium Ther Nucl Med* 1973;114:340.

Wolfson SL, Frech R, Hewitt C, et al: Radiographic diagnosis of hyaline membrane disease. *Radiology* 1969;93:339.

Pulmonary Function Testing

Cook CD, Sutherland JM, Segal S, et al: Studies of respiratory physiology in the newborn infant. III. Measurements of mechanics of respiration. *J Clin Invest* 1957;36:440.

England SJ: Current techniques for assessing pulmonary function in the newborn infant. *Pediatr Pulmonol* 1988;4:48-53.

Gerhardt T, Bancalari E: Chestwall compliance in full-term and premature infants. *Acta Paediatr Scand* 1980;69:359.

Krieger I: Studies on mechanics of respiration in infancy. *Am J Dis Child* 1963;105:439.

Lesouef PN, England SJ, Bryan AC: Passive respiratory mechanics in newborns and children. *Am Rev Respir Dis* 1984;129:552.

McCann EM, Goldman SL, Brady JP: Pulmonary function in the sick newborn infant. *Pediatr Res* 1987;21:313.

McIlroy MB, Tierney DF, Nadel JA: A new method for measurement of compliance and resistance of lungs and thorax. *J Appl Physiol* 1963;18:424.

Nelson NM, Prod'hom LS, Cherry RB, et al: Pulmonary function in the newborn infant. V. Trapped gas in the normal infant's lung. *J Clin Invest* 1963;42:1850.

Nelson NM: Neonatal pulmonary function. *Pediatr Clin North Am* 1966; 13:769.

NHLBI Workshop Summary: Assessment of lung function and dysfunction in studies of infants and children. *Am Rev Respir Dis* 1993;148:1105-1108.

Polgar G, Promadhat V: *Pulmonary Function Testing in Children: Techniques and Standards.* Philadelphia, WB Saunders Co, 1971, pp 1-273.

Chapter 4

Acute, Acquired Parenchymal Lung Disease

Hyaline Membrane Disease

Hyaline membrane disease (HMD), also called respiratory distress syndrome (RDS), causes severe progressive respiratory distress in preterm infants.

Epidemiology

It occurs in approximately 40,000 infants each year, and in about 14% of low-birth-weight infants in the United States. The incidence increases with decreasing gestational age and reaches 60% to 80% in infants born at less than 28 weeks' gestation. Numerous factors have been identified as either increasing or decreasing the risks of HMD (Tables 1 and 2).

Pathophysiology

The primary cause of HMD is surfactant deficiency, which results when the rate of use of surfactant exceeds the rate of production. Surfactant production and secretion are developmentally regulated, so the most common cause of deficiency is delivery before term (see *Surfactant* section, Chapter 2).

Lung Function

Mechanics. Insufficient surfactant at the alveolar, air-liquid interface increases surface tension and decreases lung

Table 1: Factors Increasing Risk of HMD

- Prematurity
- Male sex
- White race
- Cesarean section delivery
- Gestational diabetes
- Second-born twin
- Family history of HMD

Table 2: Factors Decreasing Risk of HMD

- Pregnancy-induced hypertension
- Chronic maternal hypertension
- Subacute placental abruption
- Maternal narcotic addiction
- Premature rupture of membranes
- Prenatal corticosteroids

compliance. As a result, the pressure required to inflate the lung is increased (Figure 1). This means that during a spontaneous inspiration, the infant must generate a large, negative intrapleural pressure to inflate its lungs. This large, negative pressure results in marked chest wall retractions and paradoxical or see-saw respirations. Overall, the work of breathing is increased.

The Laplace relationship states that the pressure (P) required to maintain an airspace at a given radius of curvature (r) is equal to twice the surface tension (T) divided by the radius ($P = 2 \times T/r$) (see *Surfactant* section, Chapter 2). At the end of exhalation, as the radius of curvature of the infant's

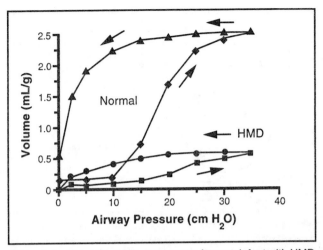

Figure 1: Lungs obtained at postmortem from an infant with HMD (lower curve) require far more pressure to achieve a given volume of inflation than do those obtained from an infant dying of a nonrespiratory cause. The arrows depict the inspiratory and expiratory limbs of the pressure volume curves. (Gribetz I: *J Clin Invest* 1959;38:2168.)

airspaces decreases, the pressure required to keep them expanded increases, and the tendency is toward collapse. The highly compliant chest wall of the premature infant is unable to resist this tendency to collapse. Therefore, the infant develops progressive atelectasis, and resting lung volume or functional residual capacity decreases. The expiratory grunt and tachypnea characteristic of the infant with HMD represent attempts to prevent lung collapse. The expiratory grunt increases end-expiratory lung volume by applying end-expiratory pressure to the lungs, while tachypnea shortens expiratory time and prevents complete emptying of the lungs during exhalation.

While total airway resistance increases only slightly in infants with HMD, regional increases in resistance may be

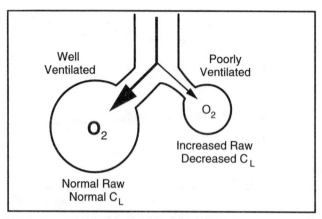

Figure 2: In infants with HMD the lung can be divided into three ventilatory compartments: (1) a well-ventilated compartment that has normal compliance and airway resistance, hence a normal to high alveolar Po_2. The bulk of the gas flow in and out of the lung occurs through this compartment; (2) an open, yet poorly ventilated compartment with decreased lung compliance and increased airway resistance. Because this compartment is severely underventilated, O_2 delivery to alveoli from the atmosphere is much less than the rate of O_2 removal by the blood, so alveolar Po_2 is markedly decreased; (3) atelectatic lung units that are not ventilated (not shown in this figure).

quite large. Airway resistance increases in infants with HMD because small airways:

- are also affected by surface tension, and their radius decreases in the face of surfactant deficiency;
- are compressed by interstitial edema (see *Pulmonary Edema* section, this chapter);
- are damaged by the large shear forces generated by attempts to expand the poorly compliant air sacs.

Despite the small increase in total airway resistance, the decrease in total lung compliance dominates measurements of pulmonary function, and the time constant for the whole lung remains very short, on the order of 0.1 seconds.

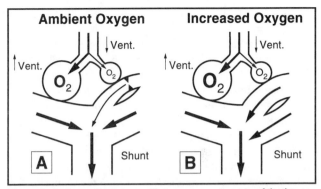

Figure 3: **A** shows the two ventilatory compartments of the lungs with HMD described in Figure 2: well-ventilated lung units in which the alveolar P_{O_2} is normal or increased, and open, severely underventilated lung units in which the alveolar P_{O_2} is markedly reduced. Blood flowing through each of these two compartments is shown by the arrows, as is blood flowing through the right-to-left shunt. **B** shows the effect of increasing the inspired oxygen tension on the lung of the infant with HMD.

Distribution of ventilation. HMD is a heterogeneous disorder with some airspaces more affected than others. This results in three distinct populations of airspaces (Figure 2).

Hypoxemia. In infants with HMD, hypoxemia is the result of right-to-left shunting of blood:
- through shunt vessels in the lung,
- past atelectatic airspaces, and
- through the ductus arteriosus and foramen ovale.

In infants with HMD, most of the right-to-left shunt occurs in the lung through vessels that have formed before formation of alveoli. Right-to-left shunting of blood past atelectatic alveoli is limited by hypoxic vasoconstriction in these lung units. Right-to-left shunt across the foramen ovale and ductus arteriosus is unusual after the first 24 hours. In fact, *left-to-right shunts* across the ductus arteriosus often complicate the later course of HMD.

Right-to-left shunting occurs because blood vessels perfusing open but poorly ventilated lung units constrict in response to the marked reduction in alveolar Po_2 (Figure 3). Poorly oxygenated blood flowing through the right-to-left shunt and past underventilated lung units mixes with well-oxygenated blood flowing through the well-ventilated portion of the lung. The Po_2 of this mixture, hence the ultimate arterial Po_2, is determined by the relative volumes of blood flowing past each compartment. Since little blood flows past the open, severely underventilated lung units, the chief contributor to arterial hypoxemia is the right-to-left shunt. *However, the magnitude of blood flow through the shunt is determined both by the extent of hypoxic vasoconstriction in the underventilated lung and by the size of the underventilated compartment relative to the rest of the lung.* With increases in Fio_2, alveolar oxygen tensions increase in both ventilated lung compartments. Blood flowing past well-ventilated lung units is nearly saturated, regardless of the Fio_2, so that increases in their alveolar Po_2 result in little change in O_2 content (see $\dot{V}_A/\dot{Q}$ section, Chapter 2). Increasing Fio_2 will have little effect on alveolar Po_2 in severely underventilated lung units until the Fio_2 becomes quite high, approaching 1.00. At this point, a nitrogen washout occurs and alveolar Po_2 increases dramatically, leading to relief of hypoxic vasoconstriction in the poorly ventilated part of the lung, increased blood flow past these now well-oxygenated lung units, decreased right-to-left shunt, and relief of arterial hypoxemia. Increasing airway pressure by administration of continuous positive air pressure (CPAP) or by intermittent mandatory ventilation (IMV) increases oxygenation in infants with HMD by improving ventilation to poorly ventilated lung units, increasing alveolar Po_2 at each Fio_2 (see *Positive Pressure Ventilatory Support*, Chapter 10).

Dead space. In infants with HMD, most of the gas flow in and out of the lung occurs in well-ventilated lung units. However, a substantial amount of the blood flows through the right-to-left shunt or past severely underventilated lung units. Therefore, the well-ventilated units are ventilated out of proportion to their perfusion and, as such, they effectively increase the total physiologic dead space in the lung. Because dead space is increased, these infants often have an increased minute ventilation with normal or only slightly reduced arterial Pco_2.

Pulmonary edema invariably complicates the course of HMD. Diversion of blood away from poorly ventilated lung units means that there will be more blood flow to normal lung units. This will result in higher vascular pressures and a higher filtration pressure (see *Pulmonary Edema* section, this chapter). In addition, overdistention of more normal lung units can injure the capillary endothelium and increase permeability to fluid and protein. The transport of interstitial fluid into airspaces (alveolar flooding) is potentiated by injury to terminal lung units from the distending pressures generated to inflate the lung. With alveolar flooding, plasma proteins enter the airspaces, further inactivating surfactant and also forming the hyaline membranes characteristic of this disorder.

Infants with HMD also develop marked peripheral edema that increases over the first 48 to 72 hours after birth and then resolves with a brisk diuresis as pulmonary function begins to improve. Interestingly, with surfactant replacement therapy, lung function often improves before the diuresis occurs, suggesting that the two are not functionally related. The etiology of this edema is not clear.

Pathology. Grossly, the lungs are poorly aerated and congested. Microscopic examination reveals diffuse atelectasis of distal airspaces and distal airways that are overdistended. The airspaces are lined with necrotic epithelium and plasma proteins. The protein lining the airspaces appears pink on microscopic sections stained with hematoxylin and eosin. The disease gets its name from this hyalinelike appearance. Injury to the airway epithelium is a universal accompaniment to HMD. Presumably, overdistended airways proximal to ar-

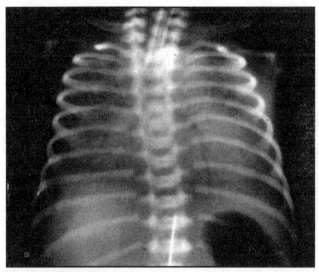

Figure 4: Chest radiograph of an infant with HMD. Lung volumes are low despite application of positive pressure through the endotracheal tube. The lungs have a homogeneous, reticular, granular appearance.

eas of collapse result in damage to airway epithelium with sloughing and exudation of plasma into the airways and airspaces.

Presentation

History. The typical history is that of a premature infant with symptoms of respiratory distress at birth. Respiratory distress increases in severity over 24 to 72 hours, then begins to resolve spontaneously. Improvement is heralded by a diuresis.

Physical examination. Infants are tachypneic, with retractions and expiratory grunting. Breath sounds are decreased bilaterally. They have cyanosis in room air, peripheral pallor, and edema.

X-ray. The chest radiograph reveals a low-volume lung (Figure 4). The lung parenchyma has a diffuse, reticular, granular, *ground-glass* appearance with air bronchograms. Occasionally, the disease process may appear worse in one lung than in the other. If the infant has already received positive pressure, the chest x-ray may appear better expanded and less granular.

Laboratory. Arterial blood gases demonstrate hypoxemia in room air that is relieved by breathing oxygen. The arterial P_{CO_2} may be normal or decreased initially but increases as the disease progresses. If the baby has retained significant fetal lung fluid in addition to having a surfactant deficiency, the P_{CO_2} may be elevated at birth.

Because infants with HMD are oliguric early in their course, serum Na^+ will decrease if fluid is not restricted until the diuresis occurs. Serum glucose should be monitored because these stressed premature infants are at risk for hypoglycemia.

Differential Diagnosis

Bacterial pneumonia, especially secondary to infection with group B streptococci, is difficult to distinguish from HMD. The clinical presentation and chest radiograph findings can be identical. Sometimes, the lungs of babies with pneumonia may initially be more compliant than those with HMD. Treatment with antibiotics of infants with abnormal radiographs and persistent or worsening oxygen requirements may be warranted until cultures are negative.

Transient tachypnea of the newborn (TTN) may present with a similar clinical picture of tachypnea, oxygen requirement, and increased work of breathing. Classically, infants with TTN will be sickest shortly after birth, with gradual improvement over hours to days. Infants with TTN will have a lower O_2 requirement (usually less than 50%) and a higher Pa_{CO_2}. The chest x-ray is helpful in differentiating TTN from HMD. Infants with TTN have a relatively high-volume lung with lacelike densities emanating from the hilum, while in-

Table 3: Effects of Antenatal Corticosteroids and Prophylactic Surfactant on the Outcome of Premature Infants

	Corticosteroids		No Corticosteroids	
	Surfactant (n = 58)	No surfactant (n = 46)	Surfactant (n = 557)	No surfactant (n = 567)
Birth weight	992 ± 200	1013 ± 226	1012 ± 284	1021 ± 281
Gest age	27.4 ± 1.8	27.5 ± 1.8	27.2 ± 2.6	27.1 ± 2.6
% Males	62%	63%	57%	53%
RDS deaths	0	6.5%	7.2%	19.6%
All deaths	0	15.2%	17.7%	24.9%
Air leaks	1.7%	13%	11%	23%
BPD	48%	55%	61%	62%
PDA	27%	22%	47%	44%
IVH	8%	9%	22%	21%

Summary data from combined prophylaxis (infants 23 to 29 weeks' gestation) and rescue (infants between 600 and 1,750 g) trials of Survanta. Jobe, et al: *Am J Obstet Gynecol* 1983;168:508.

fants with HMD have very low volume lungs with a more homogeneous appearance.

Pulmonary edema from primary cardiovascular anomalies, especially patent ductus arteriosus (PDA), may mimic HMD or complicate the course of established HMD. These infants might not have obvious symptoms of a PDA and the diagnosis may only be made by echocardiogram. Infants with obstructed anomalous pulmonary venous return may have an initial clinical course similar to HMD but fail to improve over time and usually have a fixed right-to-left shunt. *They do not improve even transiently with oxygen.* Finally, infants with congenital abnormalities of the lymphatic system, pulmonary lymphangiectasia, can mimic HMD initially and can also be distinguished by their failure to improve over time.

Aspiration pneumonia, from either meconium or amniotic fluid, may present like HMD but is unusual in premature infants and demonstrates a different radiographic appearance.

Prevention

Because HMD is a disease of premature infants, prevention of preterm delivery will prevent HMD. For those infants who are destined to deliver prematurely, however, multiple controlled trials have shown that the risk of HMD can be reduced substantially by administering corticosteroids to their mothers before delivery (Table 3). Despite these trials, prior to 1994 only 15% of eligible mothers in this country received antenatal glucocorticoids. In the spring of 1994, the National Institutes of Health convened a Consensus Conference to evaluate the role of antenatal corticosteroids in prevention of HMD. This panel recommended that:

- the benefits of antenatal administration of corticosteroids to women at risk of preterm delivery vastly outweigh the potential risks. These benefits include not only a reduction in the risk of HMD but also a substantial reduction in mortality and intraventricular hemorrhage (IVH);
- all mothers with fetuses between 24 and 34 weeks' gestation at risk of preterm delivery should be considered candidates for antenatal treatment with corticosteroids;
- the decision to use antenatal corticosteroids should not be altered by fetal race or gender or by the availability of surfactant replacement therapy;
- patients eligible for therapy with tocolytics should also be eligible for treatment with antenatal corticosteroids;

- treatment consists of two doses of 12 mg of betamethasone given IM 24 hours apart, or four doses of 6 mg of dexamethasone given IM 12 hours apart. Optimal benefit begins 24 hours after initiation of therapy and lasts 7 days;
- because treatment with corticosteroids for less than 24 hours is still associated with significant reductions in neonatal mortality, in RDS, and in IVH, antenatal corticosteroids should be given unless immediate delivery is anticipated;
- in preterm premature rupture of membranes at less than 30 to 32 weeks' gestation in the absence of clinical chorioamnionitis, antenatal corticosteroid use is recommended because of the high risk of IVH at these early gestational ages;
- in complicated pregnancies where delivery before 34 weeks' gestation is likely, antenatal corticosteroid use is recommended unless there is evidence that corticosteroids will have an adverse effect on the mother or unless delivery is imminent.

Since the Consensus Conference, the administration of antenatal corticosteroids to eligible women has increased to almost 60% in most centers, with many reporting even greater compliance.

Recent double-blind, placebo-controlled studies have not identified any additional benefit of antenatal thyroid-releasing hormone to antenatal corticosteroids used to mature the neonate's lung.

Management

HMD is a transient, self-limited disease. The stress of preterm birth rapidly matures the surfactant system so that the lung can produce adequate surfactant within 48 to 72 hours of birth. Therefore, the goal of management is to support the infant until the disease resolves without inducing further lung injury.

Surfactant. Surfactant replacement therapy directly addresses the cause of HMD, surfactant deficiency, and is now a mainstay in the early management of HMD. Multiple controlled trials have shown that surfactant replacement markedly decreases the mortality and morbidity of babies with HMD, especially small, premature babies. Surfactant replacement increases compliance and decreases resistance in surfactant-deficient lung units, thereby reducing both the distending pressures needed to inflate the lung and the work of breathing in the spontaneously breathing infant. In addition, surfactant replacement improves ventilation to open, poorly ventilated lung units and increases their alveolar Po_2. As a result, hypoxic vasoconstriction is relieved, the right-to-left shunt decreases, and overall arterial oxygenation improves.

Two types of surfactant preparations are available:
- *Survanta®* (beractant), a surfactant derived from minced calf lung with added synthetic disaturated phosphatidylcholine, and
- *Exosurf®* (colfosceril), a synthetic surfactant consisting primarily of disaturated phosphatidylcholine plus the alcohol of palmitic acid (hexadecanol).

In addition, there are now two clearly defined treatment strategies for administration of surfactant. *Prophylactic therapy* requires that the surfactant preparation be instilled in the infant's trachea soon after birth, often before a diagnosis of HMD can be established. Prophylactic therapy is frequently administered in the delivery room. *Rescue therapy* is designed to treat infants with established HMD.

Since the mid-1980s a large number of controlled trials have shown that therapy with surfactant:
- is safe;
- reduces mortality from HMD;
- decreases the incidence of pulmonary airleaks; and
- decreases the incidence of intracranial hemorrhage in small infants.

Furthermore, these studies have shown that:

- 2 to 3 doses of surfactant are superior to a single dose for both prophylaxis and rescue modes of treatment, and
- for very immature infants, <30 weeks' gestation, prophylactic therapy is superior to rescue therapy.

Administration. In our institution, all infants <30 weeks' gestation are intubated and ventilated in the delivery room and then are given *prophylactic surfactant* (see *Surfactant Administration*, Chapter 10). They receive at least two doses, with the third dose being optional.

Older infants are treated when they meet these criteria for *rescue therapy*:

- they must be intubated;
- they must have an a/A ratio of <0.22. In our institution, we consider all infants who require F_{IO_2} >0.5 to maintain Pao_2 >50 torr candidates for intubation and treatment with surfactant. Surfactant can be administered to infants who are being supported by CPAP.

Rescue therapy also consists of two doses of surfactant, with the third dose being optional.

General Support

Resuscitation. Because infants born prematurely are at high risk for developing HMD, they should be resuscitated immediately after birth. This should include expansion of the lungs with positive pressure if spontaneous respiratory efforts do not result in complete lung expansion.

Temperature control. These infants must remain in a neutral thermal environment, either on a radiant warmer or in an isolette.

IV fluids. They should be given glucose-containing IV fluids to provide some energy substrate and prevent hypoglycemia (typically 6 mg/kg/min of glucose). They are often oliguric during the first 24 to 48 hours after birth so it is our practice to restrict fluids in infants with HMD to 60 mL/kg/d. This practice may need to be modified in the very immature infant where insensible water losses may be very high.

Circulatory support. Many infants with HMD, especially infants <28 weeks' gestation, have systemic hypotension. Excessive administration of volume to treat the hypotension is usually ineffective and often worsens the lung disease. If necessary, judicious use of volume to rule out hypovolemia can be tried, but then administration of dopamine is appropriate to increase cardiac output and diminish peripheral vasodilatation.

Infection. Because of the difficulty in distinguishing HMD from bacterial pneumonia, we consider treatment of infants with HMD with antibiotics. We monitor drug levels and continue antibiotics until cultures are negative. In the severely ill or preterm infant, the lumbar puncture is often deferred until the respiratory status improves.

Respiratory therapy. Administration of oxygen, CPAP, and positive pressure ventilation still represent mainstays in the management of the infant with HMD. All of these therapies work by increasing the Po_2 in poorly ventilated lung units, relieving hypoxic vasoconstriction, and reducing the right-to-left shunt. Administration of oxygen increases the diffusion gradient for oxygen into poorly ventilated lung units (Figure 3), while CPAP and IMV increase ventilation, hence the rate of oxygen delivery to those units. Oxygen and mechanical ventilation do not cure the infant; they merely support the infant during the transient illness. These modes of support can also cause injury, so the lowest level of support should be chosen to provide adequate tissue delivery of oxygen.

Oxygen. The first level of support is supplemental oxygen (see *Oxygen* section, Chapter 10). The infant must be large and vigorous enough to be able to sustain tachypnea and an expiratory grunt to preserve functional residual capacity. Also, the infant should not have, or be at high risk for, apnea. Therefore, the candidates for supplemental oxygen alone are large prematures greater than 1,500 g.

CPAP is reserved for larger premature infants who can maintain spontaneous ventilation without apnea (see *CPAP*, Chapter 10). Typically, these infants are >1,500 g birth weight and ≥30 weeks' gestation. We begin CPAP when infants require FIO_2 >0.5 to maintain PaO_2 >50 torr. While nasal CPAP is often effective in improving oxygenation in infants with HMD, we now use endotracheal tube CPAP exclusively so that we can also administer rescue doses of surfactant at the same time.

Positive pressure ventilation (see *Positive Pressure Ventilatory Support*, Chapter 10). We intubate and ventilate from birth all infants <30 weeks' gestation. Older infants become eligible for positive pressure ventilation if they develop apnea or if they cannot maintain adequate oxygenation with an FIO_2 of 1.00 and maximum CPAP (8 to 10 cm H_2O). We do not routinely ventilate infants with increasing $PaCO_2$ in the absence of apnea or hypoxemia.

High-frequency ventilation. During high-frequency oscillatory ventilation, the infants are ventilated at very rapid rates (3,000 breaths/min) at tidal volumes less than dead-space volume. Theoretically, ventilation with low tidal volumes decreases barotrauma to the lung and results in fewer complications. Controlled trials of oscillatory ventilation for infants with HMD have not shown any consistent benefit over conventional ventilation. Moreover, three of the trials found an increased incidence of severe IVH in infants who received oscillatory ventilation. This therapy for HMD must still be considered experimental.

Extracorporeal membrane oxygenation (ECMO). Large infants with HMD who fail to respond to surfactant therapy and to mechanical ventilation may be candidates for ECMO (see *ECMO*, Chapter 10). Typically, these infants must be greater than 34 weeks' gestation and weigh more than 2,000 g.

Failure to Improve

Occasionally, infants will fail to improve with surfactant replacement therapy. These infants should be carefully evaluated for the presence of a PDA or other congenital heart disease. On the other hand, some infants will improve transiently and then deteriorate on the second or third day of therapy. This is a classic presentation for a PDA or for nosocomial pneumonia.

Outcome

HMD is a transient disease and most infants who have it recover without sequelae. Although mortality increases with decreasing gestational age, administration of antenatal corticosteroids to the mother and surfactant to the newborn can significantly improve survival (Table 3). The incidence of chronic lung disease, defined as an oxygen requirement at 28 days of age, depends heavily on gestational age and ranges from less than 10% for infants weighing more than 1,000 g at birth to nearly 50% for those between 500 and 1,000 g at birth. Severe chronic lung disease requiring supplemental oxygen for weeks to years is now rare in many neonatal intensive care units. Neurologic sequelae such as IVH are clearly associated with HMD but are substantially reduced by the administration of antenatal corticosteroids.

By Alicia A. Moïse, MD, and Thomas N. Hansen, MD

Transient Tachypnea of the Newborn
Epidemiology

Transient tachypnea of the newborn, also referred to as respiratory distress syndrome type II or as delayed clearance of the fetal lung fluid, is the most common cause of respiratory distress in newborns. A number of factors have been identified as risks for TTN (Table 4), the most prominent being premature delivery and maternal sedation.

Pathophysiology

Lung fluid is contained in airways and air sacs and is secreted by the fetal lung. The volume of liquid within the potential air spaces of fetal lambs increases from 4 to 6 mL/kg

Table 4: Risk Factors for TTN

- Premature delivery
- Maternal sedation
- Delivery by elective cesarean section
- Delayed clamping of the umbilical cord
- Maternal diabetes
- Fetal distress

body weight at midgestation to more than 20 mL/kg near term. Transepithelial chloride secretion is the chief driving force responsible for the production of this liquid in the fetal lung. As a result, fetal lung fluid has a much higher chloride concentration than does plasma, interstitial fluid, or amniotic fluid (Table 5). Secretion of fetal lung fluid appears to be hormone controlled and can be inhibited by β-adrenergic agents.

Approximately two thirds of fetal lung fluid is removed from the lung before birth, during labor. Late in gestation,

Table 5: Composition of Fetal Lung Liquid

	Lung Liquid	Interstitial Fluid	Plasma	Amniotic Fluid
Sodium mEq/L	150	147	150	113
Potassium mEq/L	6.3	4.8	4.8	7.6
Chloride mEq/L	157	107	107	87
Bicarbonate mEq/L	3	25	24	19
pH	6.27	7.31	7.34	7.02
Protein g/dL	0.03	3.27	4.09	0.10

(Bland RD: *Acta Paediatr Scand* 1983;305:12)

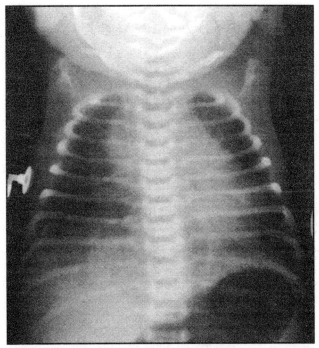

Figure 5: Chest radiograph of an infant with TTN. The lung volume is increased and there are lacelike densities emanating from the hilum. Areas of consolidation probably represent alveolar flooding.

the lung epithelium (columnar epithelial cells and type II alveolar cells) converts from chloride and fluid secretion to sodium and fluid absorption by the combined action of epithelial sodium channels and sodium, potassium-ATPase. This process increases before term and is enhanced by the presence of a large protein osmotic pressure gradient (Table 5) into the interstitium of the lung. This absorbed lung water is then cleared by the microcirculation and lymphatics. At delivery, with expansion of the lungs, the increase in pulmonary blood flow accelerates this process.

Infants born prematurely or without labor have not had sufficient time to reabsorb fetal lung fluid and, consequently, are born with excess water in their lungs. Clearance of fetal lung fluid after birth will also be delayed if the infant's lung inflation is impaired because of prematurity or the impact of maternal sedation. Any condition, such as asphyxia, that increases the rate of transvascular fluid filtration in the lung will further delay clearance of fetal lung liquid (see *Pulmonary Edema* section, this chapter).

Finally, increases in central venous pressure can impair lymphatic drainage and reabsorption of fetal lung fluid. In the newborn, venous pressure may be increased by perinatal hypoxia or by an excessive placental transfusion at delivery. Respiratory symptoms result from airway compression by fluid accumulating in the interstitium. Airway obstruction results in gas trapping, maldistribution of ventilation, and hypoxia from ventilation-perfusion mismatch.

Presentation

History. Infants with TTN usually have one or more of the risk factors listed in Table 4.

Physical examination. Tachypnea is the hallmark of the disease, with respiratory rates ranging from 60 to 120 breaths/min. In addition, expiratory grunting, chest wall retractions, nasal flaring, a barrel chest, and cyanosis in room air are frequent.

Chest x-ray. Typically, hyperinflation is seen with a sunburst pattern of linear densities emanating from the hilum. These densities represent fluid in the interstitium surrounding airways and pulmonary arteries. Occasionally, fluffy densities compatible with alveolar flooding or even pleural effusions are present (Figure 5).

Laboratory. Arterial blood gas measurements reveal hypoxemia in room air that is usually corrected by an Fio_2 <0.50. In the first hours after birth these infants frequently have hypercarbia and a mild to moderate respiratory acidosis.

Differential Diagnosis

Bacterial pneumonia is difficult to distinguish from TTN. Treatment with antibiotics of infants with abnormal chest radiographs and persistent or worsening oxygen requirements may be warranted until cultures are negative.

Aspiration pneumonia, from either meconium or amniotic fluid, may present like TTN, but will have a much longer and more complicated course.

Hyaline membrane disease (HMD), also known as respiratory distress syndrome (RDS), may initially present with TTN but worsens over time with loss of lung volume and progressive increases in oxygen requirement.

Pulmonary edema from primary cardiovascular anomalies or from congenital abnormalities of the lymphatic system (pulmonary lymphangiectasia) can mimic TTN initially. These disorders can be distinguished by typical findings of heart disease and by their failure to improve over time.

Management

TTN is a self-limited disease that usually resolves completely within 48 to 72 hours. Modest fluid restriction of 60 mL/kg/d IV is appropriate while assessing the need for supplemental oxygen. Oxygen requirements are usually highest at the onset of the disease and then decrease progressively. Infants with TTN do not usually require F_{IO_2} >0.5 or positive pressure ventilatory support. Diuretics do not alter the clinical course.

Failure to Improve

TTN is a diagnosis of exclusion. In addition, infants with increasing oxygen requirements, infants who require F_{IO_2} >0.5, or infants with any circulatory insufficiency probably do not have TTN, and the diagnosis should be reconsidered. The most common disorder confused with TTN is mild HMD. However, the possibility that the infant has pneumonia or pulmonary edema from other causes should be considered.

Table 6: Risk Factors for PPHN

- Post-term delivery
- Placental insufficiency
- Meconium staining
- Postnatal hypoxia
- Hypoglycemia
- Hypothermia
- Polycythemia
- Maternal prostaglandin inhibitors
- Bacterial pneumonia/sepsis
- Diaphragmatic hernia

Outcome

Virtually all infants with TTN recover completely without residual pulmonary disability.

By Michael E. Speer, MD, and Thomas N. Hansen, MD

Persistent Pulmonary Hypertension of the Newborn

Epidemiology

In infants with PPHN, hypoxemia results from right-to-left shunting of blood secondary to a persistently elevated pulmonary vascular resistance. The incidence of PPHN ranges from 1:425 to 1:2,000 live births. There is no known sex or race predilection. A number of risk factors for PPHN have been identified (Table 6).

Pathophysiology

Transition from intrauterine to extrauterine life requires pulmonary vascular resistance (PVR) of the fetus to decrease abruptly at birth. In infants with PPHN, this decrease does not occur. The elevated PVR diverts blood flow away from

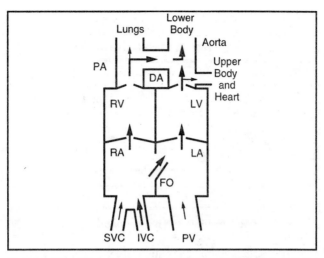

Figure 6: Circulatory pathways in an infant with PPHN. In infants with PPHN, pulmonary vascular resistance remains high after birth and pressures remain elevated in the pulmonary artery (PA), right ventricle (RV) and right atrium (RA). Poorly oxygenated blood returning from the superior vena cava (SVC) and inferior vena cava (IVC) returns to the right atrium. Because right atrial pressure is increased, much of this poorly oxygenated blood is shunted across the foramen ovale (FO) to the left atrium (LA) where it mixes with oxygenated blood returning via the pulmonary veins (PV). This atrial level right-to-left shunt reduces arterial oxygen content blood throughout the systemic arterial circulation. In addition, since pulmonary artery pressure is greater than systemic arterial pressure, poorly oxygenated blood from the pulmonary artery is shunted right-to-left through the ductus arteriosus (DA) to the descending aorta. As a result, the oxygen content, hence the Pao_2 and Sao_2 of blood obtained from below the DA, is often less than that of blood obtained from above the DA.

the pulmonary circulation through the foramen ovale and ductus arteriosus into the systemic circulation. These right-to-left shunts result in severe hypoxemia refractory to administration of oxygen (Figure 6).

Table 7: Causes of PPHN From Pulmonary Maladaptation

Transient	*Persistent*
• Hypoxia	• Meconium aspiration pneumonia
• Hypothermia	• Amniotic fluid aspiration
• Hypoglycemia	• Bacterial pneumonia
• Polycythemia	• Bacterial sepsis

There are two categories of disorders of the pulmonary vascular bed that result in PPHN, *maladaptation* and *maldevelopment*.

With *maladaptation*, the pulmonary vascular bed is structurally normal but PVR remains high. PPHN from maladaptation implies active vasoconstriction, which may be transient or persistent (Table 7).

Transient constriction usually occurs in infants who have some perinatal complication that interferes with the normal transition from intrauterine to extrauterine life. Treatment of the complication results in prompt resolution of pulmonary hypertension. While polycythemia is not associated with active constriction, it is included in this category because it is rapidly reversible with reduction of the hematocrit.

Persistent vasoconstriction is associated with more severe complications of the transition. Conditions such as bacterial pneumonia result in release of mediators, like thromboxane, that result in intense pulmonary vasoconstriction. This persistent vasoconstriction is often accompanied by evidence of plugs of platelets in the pulmonary microcirculation.

With *maldevelopment*, the pulmonary vessels are abnormal. The medial musculature is hypertrophied and extends into normally nonmuscularized arteries down to the level of the alveolus. Excessive muscularization impinges on the ves-

Table 8: Causes of PPHN From Pulmonary Maldevelopment

Maldevelopment	Underdevelopment
• Intrauterine asphyxia	• Diaphragmatic hernia
• Meconium aspiration	• Potter's syndrome
• Fetal ductal closure	• Other causes of pulmonary hypoplasia
• Congenital heart disease	

sel lumen, increasing vascular resistance. A common thread linking most cases of maldevelopment is chronically increased pulmonary blood flow in utero. Because the pulmonary and systemic circulations of the fetus are connected, conditions such as intrauterine hypoxia or asphyxia that increase systemic arterial blood pressure in the fetus will divert more blood to the lung, resulting in pulmonary vessel maldevelopment.

Presumably, fetal hypoxia and asphyxia also play a role in the vessel maldevelopment that complicates intrauterine aspiration of meconium. In experimental animals, closure of the ductus arteriosus in utero forces all of the right ventricular output through the lungs and also results in maldevelopment of pulmonary vessels. Because ductal patency in late gestation is maintained by prostaglandins, intrauterine ductal closure may occur in human pregnancies if the mother is exposed to prostaglandin synthetase inhibitors such as aspirin or indomethacin.

Finally, infants with certain types of congenital heart disease, especially those with obstructed anomalous venous drainage, may have abnormal pulmonary vessels, and pulmonary hypertension often complicates their postoperative course.

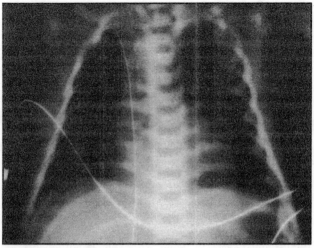

Figure 7: Chest radiograph of an infant with idiopathic PPHN. The lung fields are black, reflecting the reduced pulmonary blood flow. The heart is moderately enlarged. (Adapted from Hansen TN, Corbet AJ. In: Taeusch HW, et al, eds. *Schaffer and Avery's Diseases of the Newborn.* 5th ed. Philadelphia, WB Saunders, 1991.)

Infants with hypoplastic or *underdeveloped* lungs will have persistently elevated pulmonary vascular resistance because of the reduction in number of blood vessels per cross-sectional area of lung. In these infants, pulmonary vessels are also maldeveloped (Table 8).

A recently described rare cause of PPHN is alveolar capillary dysplasia or misalignment of lung vessels.

Presentation

History. The typical infant with PPHN is term or postterm with a history of one or more of the risk factors in Table 6.

Physical examination. The infant is cyanotic and usually tachypneic. Other signs of respiratory distress are related to the underlying lung disease. There may be a heart murmur characteristic of tricuspid insufficiency or a single S_2.

Chest radiograph. In PPHN after asphyxia or ductal closure, the lung fields are black, and the heart size is normal or increased. For other causes, the chest x-ray reflects the underlying lung disease (Figure 7).

Laboratory. Arterial blood gases reveal hypoxemia with normal $Paco_2$. Right-to-left shunting of blood across the ductus may cause the measured Sao_2 to be higher in preductal blood compared with postductal blood. Blood obtained from the right radial artery usually has a higher Sao_2 than blood from the umbilical artery, or the pulse oximeter demonstrates a differential Sao_2 between the right arm and the rest of the body. *This differential Sao_2 strongly supports a diagnosis of PPHN.* However, if the right-to-left shunt is primarily at the atrial level or if the ductus was closed in utero by exposure to prostaglandin synthesis inhibitors, there will be no Sao_2 gradient. Increasing the Fio_2 to 1.00 (the hyperoxia test) may increase Pao_2 in infants with PPHN, especially early in their course. *Infants in whom Pao_2 can never be increased, even transiently **with** hyperoxia or hyperventilation, should be carefully evaluated for cyanotic heart disease.*

Cardiac evaluation. The EKG may reveal ST segment changes compatible with subendocardial ischemia. The echocardiogram reveals normal cardiac anatomy while Doppler studies reveal right-to-left shunting across the ductus arteriosus and foramen ovale. In addition, a jet of tricuspid insufficiency can often be detected, confirming the elevated right ventricular pressures.

Differential Diagnosis

Infection is a common cause of PPHN. We treat all infants with PPHN with antibiotics until cultures are negative.

Cyanotic congenital heart disease, especially total anomalous venous return, is difficult to distinguish from PPHN. Almost all patients with PPHN will have an adequate Pao_2 at some point in their course. If they never achieve adequate oxygenation, even transiently, then the clinician should consider heart disease as a cause.

Management

PPHN is a self-limited disease and treatment is generally supportive. The goal of therapy is to lower oxygen demands and maintain oxygen delivery to the tissues until the PVR decreases.

Decrease oxygen demand. These infants must be in a neutral thermal environment to minimize oxygen consumption. If they are receiving assisted ventilation, they should be sedated with morphine sulfate (0.1 mg/kg per dose) or fentanyl (bolus of 2 to 10 µg/kg per dose). Sedation also limits additional pulmonary vasoconstriction in response to stimuli such as suctioning. Neuromuscular blockade with pancuronium bromide, 0.1 mg/kg per dose, is reserved for infants requiring extremely high ventilator pressures.

Increase oxygen delivery. Oxygen delivery is determined by the cardiac output, the arterial oxygen content, hemoglobin concentration, and Sao_2.

Cardiac output should be supported with volume replacement and dopamine at rates of infusion up to 20 µg/kg/min.

Hemoglobin concentration should be maintained at approximately 15 g/dL by transfusion with packed red cells. Higher hemoglobin concentrations may result in hyperviscosity and exacerbate right-to-left shunting.

Oxygen saturation and Pao_2 should be increased by first improving the distribution of ventilation and then by directly attempting to lower the PVR.

Improve distribution of ventilation. In infants with PPHN and parenchymal lung disease, open, underventilated lung units contribute to hypoxemia, as in HMD. Therefore, management should be similar to that of the infant with HMD (see *HMD*, this chapter).

Because of the presence of open, poorly ventilated lungs, positive end-expiratory pressure (PEEP) is often useful in improving oxygenation in infants with PPHN and parenchymal lung disease.

Ventilation. *Alkalinization, hyperventilation,* and the *avoidance of hypoxemia* using conventional ventilation techniques may reduce pulmonary artery pressures. This was first proposed as a therapy for infants with pulmonary hypertension with no associated lung disease and was based on animal studies that demonstrated sensitivity of the pulmonary vasculature to hypoxia and acidosis. Subsequently, two separate investigators reported a small number of infants with high pulmonary artery pressures who responded to a brief period of hyperventilation. Since these initial reports, the intensity of ventilation has increased, and this strategy has also been applied to infants with parenchymal lung disease with associated pulmonary hypertension, both of which may contribute to the increased incidence of chronic lung disease.

The concept of **gentle ventilation** was originally reported in a retrospective series of infants with PPHN treated with a regimen using minimal ventilator settings to maintain Pao_2 between 50 and 70 mm Hg and $PaCO_2$ between 40 and 60 mm Hg. Sedation and paralysis were avoided. All infants survived and only one developed chronic lung disease. This study's findings were supported by a second case report. Although not conclusive, the lack of randomized trials demonstrating the benefit of hyperventilation and the potential concerns of respiratory alkalosis resulting in hearing loss or development delay bring into question the role of hyperventilation for all but the most severely affected infants with PPHN.

The use of **high-frequency oscillatory** or **jet ventilation** has been suggested as therapy for infants with PPHN from a variety of causes. There has been a single, controlled trial and several uncontrolled observational trials of the effect of high-frequency ventilation on this disease. This technique acts by decreasing $PaCO_2$ and, in the case of the oscillator, is an effective tool to increase oxygenation by increasing MAP and preventing atelectasis. The use of high-frequency ventilation may prevent the need for ECMO in selected patients;

however, it is not known if there is a difference in long-term outcome in these patients.

Surfactant replacement. In many centers, infants with PPHN and parenchymal lung disease receive surfactant replacement (see *Surfactant Replacement* section, Chapter 10).

Lower PVR. If improving distribution of ventilation fails to improve oxygenation, attempts should be made to actively lower the PVR.

Induced alkalosis. Raising the pH to between 7.55 and 7.65 by inducing respiratory or metabolic alkalosis will often lower PVR and improve oxygenation. To prevent lung injury from hyperventilation, a combination of mild hyperventilation with infusion of sodium bicarbonate is preferred.

Drug therapy. The ideal drug for PPHN would lower PVR and increase oxygenation with no direct effect on the systemic circulation.

In a recently published randomized, double-blind, placebo-controlled trial, inhaled nitric oxide at 20 ppm was shown to be effective in decreasing the need for ECMO in babies ≥34 weeks with severe respiratory failure from PPHN alone or in association with meconium aspiration, pneumonia/sepsis, or RDS. Many case reports have demonstrated the effectiveness of inhaled nitric oxide in lowering PVR without affecting the systemic circulation. Nitrogen dioxide and methemoglobin levels should be monitored during nitric oxide administration (see *Nonventilatory Management* section, Chapter 10).

Nitroprusside is a pulmonary and systemic vasodilator that is given by an infusion of 1 to 5 µg/kg/min. It is rapidly cleared from the circulation if hypotension occurs. Because cyanide and thiocyanate are byproducts of its metabolism, these levels must be monitored.

Tolazoline, a nonspecific α-adrenergic blocker, is given as a loading dose of 1 to 2 mg/kg, followed by an infusion of 0.15 to 0.30 mg/kg/min. Because of its limited efficacy, long half-life, and significant side effects—including hypotension and gastric bleeding—this drug is rarely used.

Monitoring. Optimally, the Pao_2 should be maintained between 80 and 100 torr. There is no physiologic reason to maintain a higher Pao_2, and hyperoxia increases the risks of oxygen toxicity to the lungs and other organs. In severe forms of PPHN, it may be safer to maintain the Pao_2 at a lower value, 35 to 45 torr, rather than risk lung injury from excessive mechanical ventilation. Clinicians must pay strict attention to ensuring adequate oxygen delivery by supporting the circulation and maintaining an adequate hemoglobin concentration. Monitoring should include arterial lactate concentrations and acid base status. A rising arterial lactate or a progressive metabolic acidosis suggests that oxygen delivery is not adequate. After 3 to 5 days of a high concentration of oxygen ($Fio_2 > 0.50$), the PVR is no longer labile and oxygen should be weaned empirically to prevent pulmonary oxygen toxicity.

ECMO. When all other modes of therapy have failed to improve oxygenation, ECMO may be used to sustain oxygenation until the pulmonary vascular resistance falls (see *ECMO* section, Chapter 10).

Failure to Improve

Infants with PPHN should begin to improve after 3 to 5 days, even on ECMO. Any infant who fails to improve should be evaluated for cyanotic congenital heart disease or some form of irreversible PPHN, such as alveolar capillary dysplasia.

Outcome

Data on outcome of these infants are limited. It is difficult to determine whether abnormalities in developmental outcome are related to the underlying disease process or to the therapy. Mortality and need for ECMO range from 20% to 40% and the incidence of abnormal neurologic outcome ranges from 12% to 25%. High incidences of hearing impairment, cerebral infarction, and intracranial hemorrhage have been reported in several studies.

By Mary E. Wearden, MD, and Thomas N. Hansen, MD

Pulmonary Edema

Epidemiology

Pulmonary edema, defined as an increase in water content of the lung parenchyma, is a major component of many neonatal lung diseases.

Pathophysiology

In the lung, fluid filters continuously from capillaries in the alveolar septum into the alveolar interstitium (Figure 8). This filtered fluid is returned to the circulation by the pulmonary lymphatics. *Pulmonary edema occurs when the rate of fluid filtration from the microcirculation into lung tissue exceeds the rate of its removal by lymphatics.*

Fluid filtration. The rate of transvascular fluid filtration (Table 9) is governed by: (1) the balance between hydrostatic and oncotic pressures, and (2) the permeability of the capillary wall to fluid. Interstitial hydrostatic pressure (Ppmv) is similar to alveolar pressure, which is nearly equal to atmospheric pressure, and has little effect on net fluid filtration. Changes in intravascular oncotic pressures are balanced by similar changes in interstitial oncotic pressure, so the net effect of oncotic pressure on fluid filtration is also small. Therefore, the capillary hydrostatic pressure is the dominant pressure governing fluid filtration. This means that there are two basic causes of increased fluid filtration in the lung: increased capillary hydrostatic pressure and increased capillary permeability.

There are two main determinants of capillary hydrostatic pressure: left atrial pressure and pulmonary blood flow. Capillary hydrostatic pressure is always less than pulmonary artery pressure and greater than left atrial pressure. As a result, increases in left atrial pressure always increase capillary hydrostatic pressure. In addition, the pulmonary vascular bed of the neonate is fully recruited at rest, so resistance to blood flow through capillaries is fixed. Since pressure is the product of blood flow and resistance, any increase in pulmonary blood flow will directly increase capillary pressure. Simi-

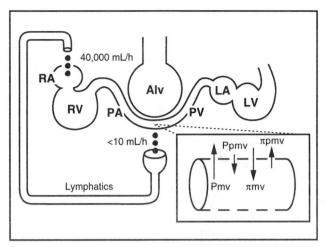

Figure 8: Blood flows from the right atrium (RA), to the right ventricle (RV), through the pulmonary artery (PA), into the capillaries in the alveolar septum. Blood returns to the heart through the pulmonary veins (PV), to the left atrium (LA), and then to the left ventricle (LV). Fluid filtration into the pulmonary interstitium occurs primarily from the capillaries in the alveolar septum (inset). Filtered fluid is transported by the pulmonary lymphatics to the thoracic duct and then returned to the central venous circulation. The rate of transvascular fluid filtration is governed by a balance between capillary and interstitial hydrostatic pressures (Pmv and Ppmv, respectively) and capillary and interstitial oncotic pressures (πmv and πpmv, respectively) and by the relative permeability of the capillary wall to fluid. Pmv tends to drive fluid out of the capillary into the interstitium, while Ppmv tends to force fluid back into the capillary. On the other hand, πmv pulls fluid into the capillary from the interstitium, while πpmv pulls fluid from the interstitium into the capillary. The net balance of these forces favors filtration of fluid from the capillary into the interstitium. However, the capillary permeability to fluid and protein is low, so that the rate of fluid filtration (<10 mL/h) is small compared to the large amount of blood circulated through the lung (>40,000 mL/h).

Table 9: Causes of Increased Transvascular Fluid Filtration

⇑ Left Atrial Pressure	⇑ Blood Flow	⇑ Permeability
• Fluid overload • Heart disease - Left-sided obstruction - Left-to-right shunt • Cardiomyopathy • Asphyxia	• Heart disease - Left-to-right shunt • ⇓ Lung vascular bed - Lung hypoplasia - Broncho-pulmonary dysplasia - Hyaline membrane disease	• Oxygen toxicity • Aspiration • Sepsis • Pneumonia • Alveolar over-distention

larly, any further decrease in the size of the vascular bed secondary to lung hypoplasia or loss of blood vessels, such as in bronchopulmonary dysplasia (BPD) or HMD, will result in a relative increase in blood flow to the remaining blood vessels and increased capillary pressure.

Capillary permeability is related to the size and number of channels available for filtration of fluid across the capillary wall. Increased capillary permeability or 'capillary leak' typically occurs secondary to conditions that injure the capillary endothelium. This injury may occur directly, by inhaled toxins such as oxygen, or indirectly, by activation of neutrophils with sepsis or pneumonia. Recently, alveolar overdistention has been shown to cause increased capillary permeability.

Lymphatic clearance. The lymphatics transport interstitial fluid through the thoracic duct into the systemic venous circulation. Recent studies found that neonate lymphatics transport fluid less efficiently than do adult lymphatics. Any impairment in lymphatic function will result in accumulation of edema fluid in the pulmonary interstitium. Impaired lymphatic function may result from primary abnormality of the lymphatics, such as in pulmonary lymphangiectasia (Chapter 6), or secondary to functional obstruction by disorders that increase systemic venous pressure, such as BPD with cor pulmonale and superior vena cava syndrome.

Sequence of edema accumulation. Fluid filters out of capillaries in the alveolar septum into the alveolar interstitium. The hydrostatic pressure in the alveolar interstitium is close to alveolar pressure (zero to slightly positive), while the pressure in the extra-alveolar interstitium is negative relative to atmospheric pressure (see *Lung and Heart Interaction* section, Chapter 2). Since these two interstitial compartments are connected, fluid in the alveolar interstitium moves along this pressure gradient into the extra-alveolar interstitium, where it can be stored in the loose connective tissue surrounding pulmonary arteries, lymphatics, and airways. Fluid entry into the alveolar spaces (alveolar flooding) occurs in the later stages of edema formation. Its presence infers that the capability of the extra-alveolar interstitium to store fluid has been exceeded or that the alveolar epithelial barrier has been damaged.

Presentation

History. There is usually a history compatible with one of the disorders listed in Table 9.

Physical examination reflects that interstitial edema compresses airways and thus increases airway resistance, resulting in an obstructive lung disease. With alveolar flooding, plasma proteins inactivate surfactant and reduce lung compliance. Both phenomena result in the creation of a population of severely underventilated lung units. Infants are often cyanotic in room air, with nasal flaring, tachypnea, and an expiratory grunt. They have barrel chests and retractions. Auscultation of the chest reveals fine rales, rhonchi, and occasional wheezes. Infants with pulmonary edema secondary to heart failure usually have an enlarged heart, gallop rhythm, and murmurs compatible with the underlying cardiac disease.

X-ray. On the chest radiograph, lung volume is usually increased. Fluid within the perivascular cuffs in the extraalveolar interstitium appears as linear densities radiating from the hilum, while alveolar flooding results in diffuse, fluffy infiltrates. In severe cases, especially with lymphatic obstruction, pleural effusions may be present. In cases secondary to heart failure, chest radiography shows the heart is enlarged.

Laboratory. The $Paco_2$ is often increased early in infants with pulmonary edema. The Pao_2 is usually reduced in room air but increases with administration of supplemental oxygen.

Differential Diagnosis

Infants with pulmonary edema secondary to *elevated left atrial pressure* typically have signs and symptoms of heart failure, including gallop rhythms, murmurs, and cardiomegaly. The exception is *obstructed anomalous pulmonary venous* drainage in which the heart size is often small. Pulmonary venous obstruction should be considered in any infant with the combination of severe progressive pulmonary edema and circulatory insufficiency. Preterm infants with *left-to-right shunts through a PDA* may develop pulmonary edema secondary to increased pulmonary blood flow in the absence of significant left ventricular failure. Any premature infant who fails to improve after surfactant therapy or who deteriorates after an initial improvement should be evaluated for a PDA even in the absence of cardiomegaly. Pulmonary edema should be expected to complicate the course of any infant with a reduced pulmonary vascular bed, (eg, pulmonary hypoplasia secondary to *diaphragmatic hernia* or loss of blood vessels secondary to *BPD*). Infants who are *ventilated with high concentrations of oxygen* for more than 2 to 3 days may develop pulmonary edema secondary to increased capillary permeability to protein. This may account for some of the later deterioration in pulmonary function that occurs in infants treated for persistent pulmonary hypertension of the newborn. Pulmonary edema secondary to *increased capillary permeability to protein* often occurs in infants with sepsis or pneumonia and may complicate episodes of massive aspiration of gastric contents. Infants with pulmonary edema secondary to lymphatic dysfunction will often have pleural effusions and may have other lymphatic anomalies such as cystic hygroma. *Pulmonary lymphangiectasia* is a primary abnormality of pulmonary lymphatics that presents as progressive pulmonary edema with no evidence for cardiac dysfunction.

Management

Treatment of pulmonary edema should be directed at correcting the etiology. For patients with PDA, this means either medical or surgical closure. For patients with self-limited diseases such as asphyxia, sepsis, or HMD, care is directed at maintaining oxygenation, decreasing fluid filtration, and waiting for spontaneous resolution. For patients with chronic pulmonary edema from BPD, heart disease that can not be corrected immediately, or lymphatic abnormalities, prolonged supportive care may be required.

Maintaining oxygenation. Oxygenation is supported by a combination of supplemental oxygen and positive airway pressure: either CPAP or IMV with PEEP (see Chapter 10). Positive airway pressure improves ventilation to open, poorly ventilated lung units and is very effective in increasing Pao_2 in patients with pulmonary edema. *However, positive airway pressure does not reduce the rate of fluid filtration in the lung nor does it reduce the rate of edema accumulation.*

Decreasing fluid filtration. Regardless of the cause of pulmonary edema, the only way to reduce the rate of fluid filtration and accumulation is to lower capillary hydrostatic pressure. Typically, this requires fluid restriction, but long-term severe fluid restriction may result in substantial growth impairment in infants. Therefore, diuretics are also used to lower circulating blood volume, hence capillary pressure. The most common diuretic used in infants with persistent pulmonary edema is furosemide (starting dose: 1 mg/kg/dose q 12 h). Aggressive diuretic therapy reduces cardiac output and renal perfusion, may result in severe metabolic disturbances such as hypokalemia and hypochloremic metabolic alkalosis, and should be used with caution. For infants with persistent pulmonary edema complicating BPD, administration of furosemide on an every-other-day regimen or substitution of a thiazide may reduce metabolic complications. The use of vasodilators to reduce capillary pressure and reduce fluid filtration in the neonate is untested. In infants with heart failure, digitalis may improve cardiac function and lower vascular pressures.

Improving lymphatic function. The only way to improve lymphatic function at the present time is to lower right atrial pressure, primarily through the use of diuretic therapy. In patients with BPD, it may also be possible to lower right atrial pressure by improving alveolar oxygenation and lowering pulmonary vascular resistance (see *BPD* section, Chapter 5).

Outcome

The outcome of patients with pulmonary edema is generally not dependent on the edema itself but rather the disease process leading to the development of pulmonary edema. Prolonged medical management of pulmonary edema in infants is complicated by malnutrition from chronic fluid restriction and bouts of circulatory insufficiency from chronic diuretic use.

By Stephen W. Welty, MD, and Thomas N. Hansen, MD

Pulmonary Hemorrhage

Epidemiology

Pulmonary hemorrhage occurs in conjunction with a number of disorders in the neonatal period, including prematurity, erythroblastosis, intracranial bleeding, asphyxia, massive aspiration, congenital heart disease, sepsis, hypothermia, PDA, and, more recently, surfactant replacement.

Pathophysiology

Pulmonary hemorrhage is most often hemorrhagic pulmonary edema. Actual blood loss is not severe. Pulmonary hemorrhage results from a sudden, large increase in capillary hydrostatic pressure that causes rupture of some capillaries and massive fluid transudation from others. The sudden increase in pressure may result from a large left-to-right shunt such as a PDA or from massive arterial and venous constriction following intracranial injury from asphyxia or intraventricular hemorrhage.

Presentation

Infants present with a history of bloody fluid in the trachea. Lung compliance decreases suddenly, and the patient usually becomes intensely cyanotic, often with signs of cardiovascular collapse. Chest radiography shows that lung fields have bilateral opacifications. The hematocrit on edema fluid is significantly lower than whole blood. Most infants have severe hypoxemia and hypercarbia.

Management

Suctioning should be performed judiciously to keep the airway clear. Positive pressure ventilation with PEEP will improve oxygenation until edema fluid clears.

Outcome

Outcome depends predominately on the cause of the pulmonary hemorrhage.

By Stephen E. Welty, MD, and Thomas N. Hansen, MD

Pleural Effusions

Epidemiology

Pleural effusions in the newborn typically accompany conditions that increase right atrial pressure or otherwise impair lymphatic function. These are congestive heart failure, chylothorax, hydrops fetalis, central venous catheter accidents, superior vena cava syndrome, and infection.

Pathophysiology

Fluid accumulates in the pleural space when the rate of fluid filtration across the pleural surfaces exceeds the rate of removal by pleural lymphatics. Filtration pressure in the parietal pleura is governed by systemic venous pressure, while filtration pressure in the visceral pleura is governed by both systemic and pulmonary venous pressures. In patients with heart failure, hydrops fetalis, or superior vena cava syndrome, elevated venous pressures increase the rate of filtration of fluid while simultaneously impairing the ability of the lymphatic system to clear this fluid. Congenital chylothorax results from intrauterine obstruction of the thoracic duct, with subsequent formation of fistulas between the intrathoracic portion of the duct and the pleural space. Acquired chylothorax occurs secondary to direct injury to the thoracic duct, usually at surgery.

Presentation

Congenital pleural effusions from hydrops fetalis or chylothorax will sometimes be detected in utero by ultrasound. A history of a central catheter (eg, for total parenteral nutrition [TPN], ECMO) is found in effusions secondary to superior vena cava syndrome or perforation of the catheter into the pleural space.

Signs and symptoms of respiratory distress are caused by compression of lung tissue by the pleural liquid and are therefore directly related to the size of the effusion. Infants with large or bilateral effusions often present with respiratory failure. The affected side of the chest may bulge, while the breath sounds over that side are decreased. Congenital bilateral effusions may be difficult to detect but should be suspected in any infant with hydrops or congenital anomalies of the lymphatic system, such as cystic hygroma. Chest radiography shows the affected side of the chest is often opacified and the heart shifted to the contralateral side. Small effusions may only be detectable by decubitus views. Laboratory examination of fluid obtained by pleurocentesis can often determine the etiology of the pleural effusion (Table 10).

Differential Diagnosis

Pleural effusions should be suspected in any infant with *hydrops fetalis* and respiratory failure in the delivery room. In these infants, emergency thoracentesis may be lifesaving. Similarly, *congenital chylothorax* should be suspected in infants with anomalies related to the lymphatic system, such as webbed neck or cystic hygroma. Pleural effusions after cardiac surgery are usually secondary to *injury to the thoracic duct*. Infants who experience sudden respiratory deterioration while receiving parenteral nutrition through a central venous catheter may well have an acquired effusion secondary to *intrapleural leakage of the IV fluids*.

Management

Thoracentesis will relieve symptoms related to pleural effusion and provide fluid to assist in differential diagnosis. Further management is related to the underlying cause. Pleural effusion secondary to leak of parenteral alimentation fluid requires removal of the central catheter. Effusions secondary to infection are rare but usually resolve with appropriate antibiotic therapy. Chylous effusions are particularly problematic and may require repeated thoracenteses and even chronic drainage via a thoracostomy tube. Chronic drainage causes substantial protein loss and may also result in lymphopenia. Once drainage is established, these infants are

Table 10: Composition of Pleural Liquid in Various Disorders

Condition	Color*	Protein Concentration†
Heart failure Hydrops fetalis SVC syndrome	Straw, clear	< Serum
Central venous catheter accident	Straw, clear or milk	< Serum
Chylothorax	Straw, clear or milky	< Serum
Infection	Turbid	> Serum

*Color of the effusion secondary to a catheter accident is milky, if lipids are being infused, but otherwise is straw-colored and clear. Color of the effusion secondary to a chylothorax is milky, if the infant is being fed milk, but otherwise is straw-colored and clear.

placed on diets containing medium-chain triglycerides rather than long-chain fats, to try to reduce thoracic duct flow. Unfortunately, oral feedings of protein and water also stimulate thoracic duct flow, so this regimen has limited utility. A variety of other techniques have been used to treat persistent chylothorax with varying degrees of success. These include direct repair of the thoracic duct, obliteration of the pleural space with sclerosing agents, pleural peritoneal shunts, and ligation of the thoracic duct below the diaphragm.

Outcome

The outcome for infants with pleural effusions is usually good. Most will resolve with treatment of the underlying disorder. While two thirds of infants with chylothorax will re-

Lipid Concentration [‡]	White Cells[§]
Low	Few
Low or high	Few
Low or high	High, mostly lymphocytes
Low	High, mostly PMNs

[†]Protein Concentration—The protein concentration when < serum is usually 2 to 4 g/dL.
[‡]Lipid Concentration—High lipid concentrations may be as much as 1,000 mg/dL.
[§]White cell counts may be as high as 10,000/mL.

spond to repeated thoracenteses alone, the mortality is still significant (approaching 15%).

By Stephen E. Welty, MD, and Thomas N. Hansen, MD

Meconium Aspiration Syndrome

Meconium staining of the amniotic fluid (MSAF) is a common problem, occurring in 9% to 20% of all deliveries. MSAF is rare before 37 weeks' gestation and common after 42 weeks' gestation (Figure 9). MSAF is neither diagnostic of fetal distress nor does it appear to be an independent predictor of subsequent neurologic morbidity in the infant. However, some of these infants subsequently develop meconium aspiration syndrome (MAS), which is associated with increased perinatal morbidity and mortality and, therefore, is a problem of particular importance in the newborn period.

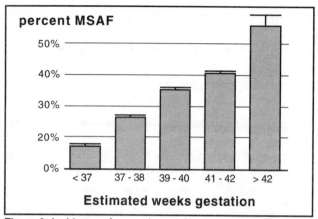

Figure 9: Incidence of meconium-stained amniotic fluid by estimated gestational age, ± 95% CI. (Used with permission, Dysart M, Graves BW, Sharp ES, et al: The incidence of meconium-stained amniotic fluid from 1980 through 1986, by year and gestational age. *J Perinatol* 1991;11:245-248).

Pathophysiology

Meconium is a viscous, greenish liquid that fills the fetal gastrointestinal tract. It is composed of gastrointestinal secretions, cellular debris, bile, pancreatic juice, mucus, blood, swallowed lanugo, and vernix. In utero, meconium passage may occur either in response to fetal hypoxia, with a transient period of hyperperistalsis and relaxation of anal sphincter tone, or as a normal, physiologic event in fetal gut maturation. Aspiration of meconium may occur in utero as the compromised, hypoxic, and acidotic fetus passes meconium and begins to gasp. More frequently, aspiration occurs with the initial breaths after delivery.

Acute large airway obstruction may occur as meconium is aspirated into the trachea. Subsequently, chemical pneumonitis and interstitial edema may obstruct smaller airways. Completely obstructed airways result in distal atelectasis. Airways with partial obstruction may allow more air to enter than to exit the distal airspace, producing air trapping. This stage of meconium aspiration is characterized by infiltration of leukocytes into the interstitial and alveolar spaces, alveolar edema, necrosis of alveolar and airway epithelia, and accumulation of proteinaceous debris in the alveoli. Alveolar injury results in surfactant inactivation and decreased lung compliance. Hypoxemia results from decreased alveolar ventilation, continued perfusion of poorly ventilated lung units, and right-to-left shunt secondary to increased pulmonary vascular resistance (PVR). PVR is increased by:

- local constriction of pulmonary vessels perfusing poorly ventilated lung units;
- global constriction of pulmonary vessels by vasoactive substances present in the aspirated meconium;
- platelet aggregation in pulmonary vessels in response to vasoactive substances in aspirated meconium; and
- maldevelopment of pulmonary vessels secondary to chronic intrauterine hypoxia.

Presentation

History. Infants with MAS are often postmature with an antenatal course frequently complicated by fetal distress. The amniotic fluid is meconium stained.

Physical examination. Tachypnea, grunting, nasal flaring, retractions, and cyanosis develop shortly after birth and progress over 12 to 24 hours. Gas-trapping results in a barrel-chested appearance. These infants often have diffuse rales and rhonchi.

X-ray. Initially, the chest radiograph may demonstrate streaky, linear densities similar to that seen in the infant with TTN. Later, the chest radiograph reveals large-volume lungs with diffuse, patchy, parenchymal infiltrates alternating with areas of overexpansion (Figure 10). Pneumomediastinum and pneumothorax are common. Occasionally, in infants with severe alveolar damage and surfactant inactivation, the chest

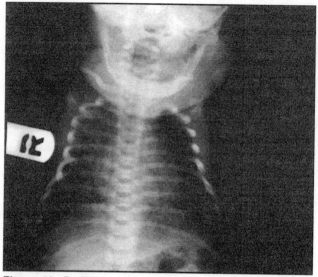

Figure 10: Radiograph of infant with MAS. The lungs are hyperinflated and dark (due to air trapping) with areas of haziness representing consolidation and alveolar edema.

radiograph may reveal low-volume lungs with homogeneous densities similar to that seen in infants with HMD.

Laboratory. Measurements of arterial blood gas tensions reveal arterial hypoxemia and hypercarbia. Infants with significant PPHN will often have a higher arterial oxygen saturation in preductal blood than in postductal blood. Spectrophotometric analysis of urine reveals an absorption at 405 nm characteristic of bile pigments present in meconium.

Differential Diagnosis

The major differential diagnoses include TTN, HMD, and bacterial pneumonia. Infants with TTN show steady improvement after birth, while those with meconium aspiration will continue to deteriorate. Infants with HMD are almost always premature, while those with meconium aspiration are term or postterm. MAS may be difficult to distinguish from bacterial pneumonia, and we often treat these infants with antibiotics, pending negative blood cultures. Aspiration of amniotic fluid with vernix caseosa may have a presentation like MAS, and the management of the two conditions is similar.

Prevention

Current recommendations for prevention of MAS call for a combined obstetric and pediatric approach to the infant born through thick or 'pea soup' meconium. This approach includes:

- Immediate suctioning of the infant's nasopharynx by the obstetrician, as the head appears on the perineum or abdomen and before delivery of the body;
- Postdelivery visualization of the vocal cords by laryngoscopy and direct suctioning of the trachea with an endotracheal tube, if possible before stimulating the infant or applying positive pressure ventilation. Universal precautions require that this suctioning be performed using a device that can be interposed between the endotracheal tube and the suction source.

Unfortunately, some infants born through thick meconium-stained fluids will develop MAS despite adequate delivery room management.

Performance of these measures in infants with thin MSAF is controversial because term infants with thin MSAF without evidence of fetal distress or compromise have limited potential for respiratory morbidity.

In addition to early clearing of the trachea, recent data suggest that intrapartum amnioinfusion may benefit infants with MSAF, possibly by diluting the meconium, by reducing its toxicity, and by correcting the oligohydramnios often associated with MSAF. Amnioinfusion may also reduce the risk of cord compression and acidemia, both of which could ultimately result in antepartum aspiration. More studies are under way to determine if this technique will enhance a favorable outcome in labors complicated by MSAF.

Management

Symptomatic infants with meconium suctioned from their trachea should be given chest physiotherapy and warmed, humidified oxygen to breathe.

Although there is no clear evidence that infection contributes to the pathogenesis of MAS, meconium is known to enhance bacterial growth by reducing host resistance. In addition, it is often difficult to distinguish MAS from other forms of pneumonia. Therefore, treatment of those infants with antibiotics should be considered pending negative blood cultures.

Corticosteroids have not been shown to play a role in the acute phase of MAS and in one study prolonged the requirement for supplemental oxygen. As a result, they are not recommended.

Tracheal lavage may result in deterioration in lung function and is not recommended.

MAS is a self-limited disease, and the goals of respiratory therapy are similar to those for PPHN—to lower oxygen demands while maintaining oxygen delivery to the tissues (see *PPHN* section, this chapter).

Clinical studies have shown that surfactant inactivation contributes to the morbidity and potential mortality of MAS. Meconium in the alveoli can injure type II alveolar epithelial cells and interfere with surfactant production. Surfactant replacement therapy, if started within 6 hours after birth, has been shown to improve oxygenation and reduce the severity of pulmonary morbidity in some cases.

Decrease oxygen demand. These infants must be in a neutral thermal environment to minimize oxygen consumption. If they are receiving assisted ventilation, they should be sedated with morphine sulfate (0.1 mg/kg per dose) or fentanyl (bolus of 2 to 10 μg/kg per dose or continuous infusion of 1 to 5 μg/kg/h). Sedation also limits additional pulmonary vasoconstriction in response to stimuli such as suctioning. Neuromuscular blockade with pancuronium bromide (0.1 mg/kg per dose) is reserved for infants requiring extremely high ventilator pressures.

Increase oxygen delivery. Oxygen delivery is determined by the cardiac output and the arterial oxygen content, ie, hemoglobin concentration and Sao_2.

Cardiac output should be supported with volume replacement and dopamine (at infusion rates of up to 20 μg/kg/min).

Hemoglobin concentration may need to be maintained at approximately 15 g/dL by transfusion with packed red cells if oxygen content is poor or if there is evidence of PPHN. Higher hemoglobin concentrations may result in hyperviscosity and exacerbate right-to-left shunting.

Oxygen saturation and Pao_2 should be increased by first improving the distribution of ventilation and then by directly attempting to lower the PVR.

Improve distribution of ventilation. In infants with MAS, open, underventilated lungs contribute to hypoxemia, and management should be similar to that of the infant with HMD (see *HMD* section, this chapter).

Surfactant replacement. Meconium in the alveoli can injure type II alveolar epithelial cells and interfere with surfactant production. In addition, meconium and edema fluid may inactivate surfactant in distal airways and alveoli. Since surfactant-deficient lung units contribute to the hypoxemia associated with MAS, therapy with surfactant may improve oxygenation (see *Surfactant Administration* section, Chapter 10).

Oxygen and ventilation. The approach to oxygen administration and ventilation is similar to that used for HMD (see *Oxygen Use and Monitoring*, Chapter 10). *Because of the presence of open, poorly ventilated lung units, judicious application of CPAP (4 to 7 cm H_2O) is often useful in improving oxygenation in infants with MAS.* Mechanical ventilation should be reserved for infants with apnea from birth asphyxia or for those who cannot maintain their Po_2 >50 mm Hg in 100% oxygen. Again, judicious use of PEEP (4 to 7 cm H_2O) may improve oxygenation. For aggressive mechanical ventilation in the large, vigorous newborn, neuromuscular blockade may optimize ventilatory support and decrease the chance of air leak. Because MAS is characterized by airway obstruction, particular attention must be paid to inspiratory time and ventilator rate to prevent unintentional PEEP that would exacerbate gas trapping and alveolar rupture.

Lower pulmonary vascular resistance (PVR). Some infants with severe MAS will also have PPHN. Therefore, if improving distribution of ventilation fails to improve oxygenation, attempts should be made to actively lower the PVR:

- *Induced alkalosis.* Raising the pH to 7.55 or greater by inducing respiratory or metabolic alkalosis will often lower PVR and improve oxygenation. Infants with MAS have an increased airway resistance and prolonged respiratory time constant. Therefore, rapid-rate ventilation may result in gas trapping, lung overdistention, and air block. To prevent lung injury from hyperventilation, a combination of mild hyperventilation with infusion of sodium bicarbonate is preferred.

- *Drug therapy*, including the use of nitric oxide, is similar to that described for the infant with PPHN.

- *Tolazoline*, a nonspecific α-adrenergic blocker, is given as a loading dose of 1 to 2 mg/kg followed by an infusion of 0.15 to 0.30 mg/kg/min. Because of its limited efficacy, long half-life, and significant side effects (including hypotension and gastric bleeding), this drug is rarely used.

- *Nitroprusside* is a pulmonary and systemic vasodilator that is given as an infusion at 1 to 5 µg/kg/min. It is rapidly cleared from the circulation should hypotension occur. Cyanide and thiocyanate are byproducts of its metabolism, and levels must be monitored.

- *Nitric oxide.* In several case reports, inhalation of nitric oxide at 20 to 80 ppm decreased PVR without affecting the systemic circulation (see *Nonventilatory Management* section, Chapter 10).

High-frequency ventilation. A single, controlled trial (and several uncontrolled observational trials) has suggested that high-frequency oscillatory ventilation at rates up to 3,000 breaths/min may be effective in improving oxygenation, thereby preventing the need for subsequent ECMO in infants with MAS and PPHN. While these reports are encouraging, this therapy must still be considered experimental.

ECMO. When all other modes of therapy have failed to improve oxygenation, ECMO can be used to sustain oxygenation (see *ECMO*, Chapter 10). In fact, since the advent of ECMO, the mortality from MAS is now quite low in most centers.

Monitoring. Optimally, the Pao_2 should be maintained between 80 and 100 torr. There is no physiologic reason to maintain a higher Pao_2, and hyperoxia increases the risks of oxygen toxicity to the lungs and other organs. In severe forms of MAS, it may be safer to maintain the Pao_2 at a lower value (35 to 45 torr) rather than risk lung injury from excessive mechanical tissue ventilation. Strict attention must be paid to insuring adequate oxygen delivery by supporting the circulation and maintaining an adequate hemoglobin concentration. Monitoring should then include arterial lactate concentrations and acid-base status. A rising arterial lactate or a progressive metabolic acidosis suggests that oxygen delivery is inadequate. After 3 to 5 days of high concentrations of oxygen ($Fio_2 > 0.50$), the PVR is no longer labile, and oxygen should be weaned empirically to prevent pulmonary oxygen toxicity.

Failure to Improve

Infants with MAS may deteriorate for 12 to 24 hours after birth but should begin to improve after 3 to 5 days—even when on ECMO. Any infant who fails to improve should be evaluated for cyanotic congenital heart disease or for a form of irreversible PPHN such as alveolar capillary dysplasia. Because meconium must ultimately be cleared from the lung by phagocytes, respiratory symptoms may persist for weeks after birth.

For those infants with MAS with profound hypoxia and PPHN, ECMO may be appropriate when conventional strategies fail.

Outcome

Symptoms related to MAS may persist for days to weeks. In the past, mortality for infants with MAS was as high as 30%. However, with the advent of a gentler approach to ventilation and, for severe cases, the availability of ECMO, mortality is now less than 10% and in some centers approaches zero. Infants with MAS are at increased risk for complications of mechanical ventilation, including air block and bronchopulmonary dysplasia.

By Karen E. Johnson, MD, Timothy R. Cooper, MD, and Thomas N. Hansen, MD

Pneumonia
Epidemiology

Pneumonia can be caused by bacterial, viral, spirochetal, protozoan, and fungal pathogens. The pneumonic process may begin before, during, or after delivery. The infant may be infected transplacentally, via infected amniotic fluid, after colonization at delivery, and nosocomially. Nosocomial infections, in many instances, can be traced to poor handwashing and overcrowding. The most common organisms associated with each route of infection are listed in Table 11.

The preterm infant is much more prone to infection than the term infant. The reasons relate to an immature immune system coupled with a lack of protective maternal antibodies.

Pathophysiology

Congenital pneumonia is not an infrequent finding at autopsy; 15% to 38% of stillborn infants have evidence of pulmonary inflammation. In most of these pneumonias, infiltration of alveoli or destruction of bronchopulmonary tis-

Table 11: Common Organisms Associated With Neonatal Pneumonia

Transplacental
- Rubella
- Cytomegalovirus
- Herpes simplex virus
- Adenovirus
- Mumps virus
- *Toxoplasma gondii*
- *Listeria monocytogenes*
- *M tuberculosis*
- *Treponema pallidum*

Amniotic Fluid
- Cytomegalovirus
- Herpes simplex virus
- Enteroviruses
- Genital mycoplasma
- *L monocytogenes*
- *Chlamydia trachomatis*
- *M tuberculosis*
- Group B streptococci (GBS)
- *Escherichia coli*
- *Haemophilus influenzae* (nontypable)

At Delivery
- GBS
- *E coli*
- *Staphylococcus aureus*
- *Klebsiella* sp
- Other streptococci
- *H influenzae* (nontypable)
- *Candida* sp
- *C trachomatis*

Nosocomial
- *S aureus*
- *S epidermidis*
- GBS
- *Klebsiella* sp
- *Enterobacter*
- *Pseudomonas*
- Influenza virus
- Respiratory syncytial virus
- Enteroviruses

sue is rare, bacteria are seen infrequently, and cultures are often negative. Aspiration or ingestion of infected amniotic fluid appears to be the most frequent cause of bacterial pneumonia. Those infections occurring during and after the birth process have findings similar to those pneumonias seen in older children. The lungs contain areas of cellular exudate with vascular congestion, hemorrhage, and necrosis.

Presentation

History. Infants who have congenital pneumonia are often critically ill at delivery or may be stillborn. The mother may give a history of an infectious process preceding delivery or may exhibit signs and symptoms of chorioamnionitis.

Physical examination. In infants who acquire their disease after birth, the signs and symptoms are frequently those of systemic infection: lethargy, poor feeding, fever, and respiratory distress or apnea. Rales and changes in the quality of the breath sounds may or may not be present.

Chest radiograph. Changes may mimic those of HMD in instances of early bacterial pneumonia, particularly these due to group B streptococci, or be nonspecific, streaky densities or confluent opacities. Abscess cavities can be seen in staphylococcal disease but can also be found in pneumonia caused by *E coli* and *K pneumoniae*.

Laboratory. Cultures of the gastric contents, throat, and nasopharynx are unrevealing or inaccurate. Direct tracheal aspiration via laryngoscopy with gram stain and culture of the resulting material can be helpful. Bacteremia and meningitis often are found in infants with pneumonia, and cultures of blood and CSF are recommended. Direct (arterial blood gas) or indirect (pulse oximetry or transcutaneous oxygen) assessment of oxygenation should be undertaken.

Differential Diagnosis

HMD, TTN, meconium aspiration, lung hypoplasia, pulmonary edema and hemorrhage, and congenital heart disease are relatively common conditions to consider in patients with neonatal pneumonia.

Management and Outcome

Obviously, prompt institution of antimicrobials is crucial. For early-onset disease, a penicillin and an aminoglycoside are usually recommended. For infection acquired in the hospital, a penicillinase-resistant penicillin or vancomycin and an aminoglycoside or third-generation cephalosporin are appropriate. Many neonatal ICUs have infections caused by *S epidermidis* or methicillin-resistant *S aureus*, requiring vancomycin. If infection by *Ureaplasma urealyticum* or *Chlamydia trachomatis* is suspected, erythromycin is the preferred antibiotic. Other supportive measures include cardiopulmonary management, fluids, and nutritional support.

In the British Perinatal Mortality Study, pneumonia was considered the cause of death in 5.5% of stillborn and neonatal deaths. The overall mortality of sepsis ranges from 5% to 10% in the term infant, to as high as 67% in the neonate <1,500 g. Infants born with fulminant group B streptococcal infection suffer a 50% mortality. Pneumonia is still a fatal complicating factor in infants with underlying congenital heart disease, CNS malformations, and anomalies of the gastrointestinal tract.

By Michael E. Speer, MD, and Leonard E. Weisman, MD

Suggested Reading

Hyaline Membrane Disease

Avery ME, Mead J: Surface properties in relation to atelectasis and hyaline membrane disease. *Am J Dis Child* 1959;97:517.

Ballard RA, Ballard PL, Boardman RC, et al: Antenatal thyrotropin releasing hormone for the prevention of chronic lung disease in the preterm infant. *Pediatr Res* 1997;41:1461A. Abstract.

Chu J, Clements JA, Cotton EK, et al: Neonatal pulmonary ischemia: clinical and physiological studies. *Pediatrics* 1967;40:709.

Corbet AJS, et al: Ventilation-perfusion relationships as assessed by aA.DN$_2$ in hyaline membrane disease. *J Appl Physiol* 1974;36:74.

Fujiwara T, Chida S, Watabe Y, et al: Artificial surfactant therapy in hyaline membrane disease. *Lancet* 1980;12:55.

Gluck L, Kulovich MV: Lecithin-sphingomyelin ratios in amniotic fluid in normal and abnormal pregnancy. *Am J Obstet Gynecol* 1973;115:539.

Gregory GA, Kitterman JA, Phibbs RH, et al: Treatment of idiopathic respiratory distress syndrome with continuous airway pressure. *N Engl J Med* 1971;284:1333.

Gribetz I, Frank NR, Avery ME: Static volume pressure relations of excised lungs of infants with hyaline membrane disease: newborn and stillborn infants. *J Clin Invest* 1959;38:2168.

Hallman M, Teramo K: Measurement of the lecithin-sphingomyelin ratio and phosphatidylglycerol in amniotic fluid: an accurate method for the assessment of fetal lung maturity. *Br J Obstet Gynecol* 1981;88:806.

Hansen TN, Corbet AJS, Kenny JD, et al: Effects of oxygen and constant positive pressure breathing on a-ADCO$_2$ in hyaline membrane disease. *Pediatr Res* 1979;13:1167.

Hansen TN, Corbet AJS: Disorders of the transition. In: Ballard R, Taeusch W, eds. *Schaffer's Diseases of the Newborn*. Philadelphia, WB Saunders Co, 1991, pp 498-504.

Horbar JD, Soll RF, Sutherland JM, et al: A multicenter, randomized, placebo-controlled trial of surfactant therapy for respiratory distress syndrome. *N Engl J Med* 1989;320:959.

Horbar JD, Wright LL, Soll R, et al: A multicenter, randomized trial comparing two surfactants for the treatment of neonatal respiratory distress syndrome. *J Pediatr* 1993;123:757.

Jobe AH: Pulmonary surfactant therapy. *N Engl J Med* 1993;328:861.

Jobe AH, Mitchell BR, Gunkel JH: Beneficial effects of the combined use of prenatal corticosteroids and postnatal surfactant on preterm infants. *Am J Obstet Gynecol* 1993;168:508.

Kattwinkel J, Bloom BT, Delmore P, et al: Prophylactic administration of calf lung surfactant extract is more effective than early treatment of respiratory distress syndrome in neonates of 29 through 32 weeks' gestation. *Pediatrics* 1993;92:90.

Kendig JW, Notter RH, Cox C, et al: A comparison of surfactant as immediate prophylaxis and as rescue therapy in newborns of less than 30 weeks' gestation. *N Engl J Med* 1991;324:865.

Liechty EA, Donovan E, Purohit D, et al: Reduction of neonatal mortality after multiple doses of bovine surfactant in low birth weight neonates with respiratory distress syndrome. *Pediatrics* 1991;88:19.

Liggins GC, Howie RN: A controlled trial of antepartum glucocorticoid treatment of prevention of the respiratory distress syndrome in premature infants. *Pediatrics* 1972;50:515.

Long W, Corbet A, Cotton R, et al: A controlled trial of synthetic surfactant in infants weighing 1250 g or more with respiratory distress syndrome. *N Engl J Med* 1991;325:1696.

Long W, Thompson T, Sundell H, et al: Effects of two rescue doses of a synthetic surfactant on mortality rate and survival without bronchopulmonary dysplasia in 700- to 1350-gram infants with respiratory distress syndrome. *J Pediatr* 1991;118:595.

NIH Consensus Development Panel Effect of Corticosteroids for Fetal Maturation on Perinatal Outcomes: Effect of corticosteroids for fetal maturation on perinatal outcomes. *JAMA* 1995;273:413-418.

Nilsson R, Grossmann G, Robertson B: Lung surfactant and the pathogenesis of neonatal bronchiolar lesions induced by artificial ventilation. *Pediatr Res* 1978;12:249.

OSIRIS Collaborative Group: Early versus delayed neonatal administration of a synthetic surfactant - the judgment of OSIRIS. *Lancet* 1992;340:1363.

Richardson P, Pace WR, Valdes E, et al: Time dependence of lung mechanics in preterm lambs. *Pediatr Res* 1992;31:276.

Shapiro DL, Notter RH, Morin III, et al: Double-blind, randomized trial of a calf lung surfactant extract administered at birth to very premature infants for prevention of respiratory distress syndrome. *Pediatrics* 1985;76:593.

Soll RF, Hoekstra RE, Fangman JJ, et al: Multicenter trial of single-dose modified bovine surfactant extract (Survanta®) for prevention of respiratory distress syndrome. *Pediatrics* 1990;85:1092.

Wright LL, Verter J, Stevenson DK, et al: Increased antenatal glucocorticoid use decreases mortality and morbidity in the NICHD Neonatal Research Network's very low birth weight infants. *Pediatr Res* 1997;41:1269A. Abstract.

Transient Tachypnea of the Newborn

Avery ME, Gatewood OB, Brumley G: Transient tachypnea of the newborn: possible delayed resorption of fluid at birth. *Am J Dis Child* 1966;111:380.

Bland RD: Formation of fetal lung liquid and its removal near birth. In: Polin RA, Fox WW, eds. *Fetal and Neonatal Physiology*. Philadelphia, WB Saunders Co, 1992, pp 782-789.

Hansen TN, Corbet A: Disorders of the transition. In: Taeusch HW, Ballard RA, Avery ME, eds. *Diseases of the Newborn*, 6th ed. Philadelphia, WB Saunders Co, 1991, pp 504-505.

Krauss AN, Auld PAM: Pulmonary gas trapping in premature infants. *Pediatr Res* 1971;5:10.

Sundell H, Garrott J, Blankenship WJ: Studies on infants with type II respiratory distress syndrome. *J Pediatr* 1971;78:754.

Persistent Pulmonary Hypertension of the Newborn

Auten RL, Notter RH, Kendig JW, et al: Surfactant treatment of full-term newborns with respiratory failure. *Pediatrics* 1991;87:101-107.

Ballard RA, Leonard CH: Developmental follow-up of infants with persistent pulmonary hypertension of the newborn. *Clin Perinatol* 1984;11:737.

Bartlett RH, Roloff DW, Cornell RG, et al: Extracorporeal circulation in neonatal respiratory failure: a prospective randomized study. *Pediatrics* 1985;76:479.

Clark RH, Yoder BA, Sell MS: Prospective, randomized comparison of high-frequency oscillation and conventional ventilation in candidates for extracorporeal membrane oxygenation. *J Pediatr* 1994;124:447-454.

Drummond WH, Gregory GA, Heymann MA, et al: The independent effects of hyperventilation, tolazoline and dopamine on infants with persistent pulmonary hypertension. *J Pediatr* 1981;98:603.

Dworetz AR, Moya FR, Sabo B, et al: Survival of infants with persistent pulmonary hypertension without extracorporeal membrane oxygenation. *Pediatrics* 1989;84:1-6.

Geggel RL, Reid LM: The structural basis of PPHN. *Clin Perinatol* 1984;11:525-549.

Gersony WM, Duc GV, Sinclair JC: "PFC" syndrome (persistence of the fetal circulation). *Circulation* 1969;39(suppl):III-87.

Hansen TN, Gest AL: Oxygen toxicity and other ventilatory complications of treatment of infants with persistent pulmonary hypertension. *Clin Perinatol* 1984;11:653.

Hansen TN, Corbet AJS: Disorders of the transition. In: Ballard R, Taeusch W, eds. *Schaffer's Diseases of the Newborn*. Philadelphia, WB Saunders Co, 1991, pp 506-509.

Hendricks-Munoz KD, Walton JP: Hearing loss in infants with persistent fetal circulation. *Pediatrics* 1988;81:650.

Hickey PR, Hansen DD, Wessel DL, et al: Blunting of stress responses in the pulmonary circulation of infants by fentanyl. *Anesth Analg* 1985;64:1137.

Kinsella JP, Neish SR, Shaffer E, et al: Low-dose inhalational nitric oxide in persistent pulmonary hypertension of the newborn. *Lancet* 1992;340:819-820.

Levin DL, Heymann MA, Kitterman JA, et al: Persistent pulmonary hypertension of the newborn infant. *J Pediatr* 1976;89:626.

Morin FC III: Ligating the ductus arteriosus before birth causes persistent pulmonary hypertension in the newborn lamb. *Pediatr Res* 1989;25:245.

Naeye RL, Schochat SJ, Whitman V, et al: Unsuspected pulmonary vascular abnormalities associated with diaphragmatic hernia. *Pediatrics* 1976;58:902.

O'Rourke PP, Crone RK, Vacanti JP, et al: Extracorporeal membrane oxygenation and conventional medical therapy in neonates with persistent pulmonary hypertension of the newborn: a prospective randomized study. *Pediatrics* 1989;84:957-963.

Roberts JD, Polaner DM, Lang P, et al: Inhaled nitric oxide in persistent pulmonary hypertension of the newborn. *Lancet* 1992;340:818-819.

Schreiber MD, Heymann MA, Soifer SJ: Increased arterial pH, not decreased $PaCO_2$, attenuates hypoxia-induced pulmonary vasoconstriction in newborn lambs. *Pediatr Res* 1986;20:113.

Wilcox DT, Glick PL, Karamanoukian H, et al: Pathophysiology of congenital diaphragmatic hernia. V. Effect of exogenous surfactant therapy on gas exchange and lung mechanics in the lamb congenital diaphragmatic hernia model. *J Pediatr* 1994;124(2):289-292.

Wung JT, James LS, Kilchevsky E, et al: Management of infants with severe respiratory failure and persistance of the fetal circulation, without hyperventilation. *Pediatrics* 1985;76:488.

Pulmonary Edema

Albertine KH: Ultrastructural abnormalities in increased-permeability pulmonary edema. *Clin Chest Med* 1985;6:345.

Bland RD, Hansen TN: Neonatal lung edema. In: Said SI, ed. *The Pulmonary Circulation and Acute Lung Injury*. Mount Kisco, NY, Futura Publishing Co, p 225, 1985.

Brigham KL, Woolverton W, Blake L, et al: Increased sheep lung vascular permeability caused by *Pseudomonas* bacteremia. *J Clin Invest* 1974;54:792.

Carlton DP, Cummings JJ, Scheerer RG, et al: Lung overexpansion increases pulmonary microvascular protein permeability in young lambs. *J Appl Physiol* 1990;69:577-583.

Drake R, Giesler M, Laine G, et al: Effect of outflow pressure on lung lymph flow in unanesthetized sheep. *J Appl Physiol* 1985;58:70.

Fein A, Grossman RF, Jones JG, et al: The value of edema fluid protein measurement in patients with pulmonary edema. *Am J Med* 1979;67:32.

Feltes TF, Hansen TN: Pulmonary edema. In: Garson AJ, Bricker JT, McNamara DG, eds. *The Science and Practice of Pediatric Cardiology*. Philadelphia, Lea and Febiger, 1990, pp 386-400.

Johnson, SA, Vander Straten MC, Parallada JA, et al: Thoracic duct function in fetal, newborn, and adult sheep. *Lymphology* 1996;29:50-56.

Staub NC, Nagano H, Pearce ML: The sequence of events during fluid accumulation in acute pulmonary edema. *Jap Heart J* 1967;8:683-689.

Staub NC: The pathogenesis of pulmonary edema. *Prog Cardiovasc Dis* 1980;33:53-80.

Pulmonary Hemorrhage

Cole VA, Normand CS, Reynolds EOR, et al: Pathogenesis of hemorrhagic pulmonary edema and massive pulmonary hemorrhage in the newborn. *Pediatrics* 1973;51:175.

Malik AB: Mechanisms of neurogenic pulmonary edema. *Circ Res* 1985;57:1.

Rowe S, Avery ME: Massive pulmonary hemorrhage in the newborn. II. Clinical considerations. *J Pediatr* 1966;69:12.

Pleural Effusions

Chernick V, Reed MH: Pneumothorax and chylothorax in the neonatal period. *J Pediatr* 1970;76:624.

Chervenak FA, Isaacson G, Blacemore KJ, et al: Fetal cystic hygroma: cause and natural history. *N Engl J Med* 1983;309:822.

Miserocchi G: Pleural pressures and fluid transport. In: Crystal RG, West JB, Barnes PJ, et al, eds. *The Lung*. New York, Raven Press Ltd, 1991, p 885.

Rodeck CH, Fisk NM, Fraser DI, et al: Long-term in utero drainage of fetal hydrothorax. *N Engl J Med* 1988;319:1135.

Smeltzer DM, Stickler GB, Fleming RE: Primary lymphatic dysplasia in children: chylothorax, chylous ascites, and generalized lymphatic dysplasia. *Eur J Pediatr* 1986;145:286.

Stringel G, Mercer S, Bass J: Surgical management of persistent postoperative chylothorax in children. *Can J Surg* 1984;27:543.

Wiener-Kronish JP, Berthiaume Y, Albertine KH: Pleural effusions and pulmonary edema. *Clin Chest Med* 1985;6:509.

Meconium Aspiration Syndrome

Al-Mateen KB, Dailey K, Grimes MM, et al: Improved oxygenation with exogenous surfactant administration in experimental meconium aspiration syndrome. *Pediatr Pulmonol* 1994;17:75-80.

Carson BS, Losey RW, Bowes WA, et al: Combined obstetric and pediatric approach to prevent meconium aspiration syndrome. *Am J Obstet Gynecol* 1976;126:712.

Davis RO, Philips JB, Haris BA, et al: Fatal meconium aspiration syndrome occurring despite airway management considered appropriate. *Am J Obstet Gynecol* 1985;151:731.

Desmond MM, Moore J, Lindley JE, et al: Meconium staining of the amniotic fluid: a marker of fetal hypoxia. *Obstet Gynecol* 1957;9:91.

Findlay, RD, Taeusch HW, Walther FJ: Surfactant replacement therapy for meconium aspiration syndrome. *Pediatrics* 1996;97:48-52.

Fox WW, Berman LS, Downes JJ, et al: The therapeutic application of end-expiratory pressure in the meconium aspiration syndrome. *Pediatrics* 1975;56:214.

Fox WW, Gewitz MH, Dinwiddie R, et al: Pulmonary hypertension in the perinatal aspiration syndromes. *Pediatrics* 1977;59:205.

Gregory GA, Gooding CA, Phibbs RH, et al: Meconium aspiration in infants - a prospective study. *J Pediatr* 1970;85:848.

Khammash H, Perlman M, Wojtulewicz J, et al: Surfactant therapy in full term neonates with severe respiratory failure. *Pediatrics* 1993;92:135-139.

Matthews TG, Warshaw JB: Relevance of the gestational age distribution of meconium passage in utero. *Pediatrics* 1979;64:30.

Park KH, Bae CW, Chung SJ: In vitro effect of meconium on the physical surface properties and morphology of exogenous pulmonary surfactant. *J Korean Med Science* 1996;11:429-436.

Rubin BK, Tomkiewicz RP, Patrinos ME, et al: The surface and transport properties of meconium and reconstituted meconium solutions. *Pediatr Res* 1996;40:834-838.

Tran N, Lowe C, Sivieri EM, et al: Sequential effects of acute meconium obstruction on pulmonary function. *Pediatr Res* 1980;14:34.

Usta IM, Mercer BM, Aswad NK, et al: The impact of a policy of amnioinfusion for meconium-stained amniotic fluid. *Obstet Gynecol* 1995;85:237-241.

Wiswell TE, Henley MA: Intratracheal suctioning, systemic infection, and the meconium aspiration syndrome. *Pediatrics* 1992;89:203-206.

Pneumonia

Hansen TN, Corbet AJS: Neonatal pneumonias. In: Ballard R, Taeusch W, eds. *Schaffer's Diseases of the Newborn*. Philadelphia, WB Saunders Co, 1991, p 527.

Klein JO: Bacterial infections of the respiratory tract. In: Remington JS, Klein JO, eds. *Infectious Diseases of the Fetus and Newborn Infant*. 4th ed. Philadelphia, WB Saunders Co, 1995, pp 891-908.

Stoll BA, Weisman LE, eds. Infections in perinatology. *Clinics in Perinatology* 1997;24:1-283.

Chapter 5

Subacute and Chronic Acquired Parenchymal Lung Diseases

Air Block
Epidemiology

Air block is far more common in the newborn period than at any other period of life. Although the observed frequency appears to be decreasing, reports of air block vary with the underlying lung disease as well as methods of resuscitation and ventilation (Table 1). Besides those with acute lung disease, infants with hypoplastic lungs, diaphragmatic hernias, and renal anomalies have a high incidence of air block.

In mature infants, air block is usually manifested by a *pneumomediastinum* or a *pneumothorax*. In the small, less than 1,500-g, premature infants, *pulmonary interstitial emphysema (PIE)* is more common.

Pathophysiology

PIE and pneumothoraces occur less as a consequence of high transalveolar pressures than because of abnormal distribution of gas and subsequent alveolar overdistention. Therefore, the normal lung, evenly ventilated and constrained by the thorax, will rarely develop air block. However, with disease (eg, hyaline membrane disease [HMD] with microatelectasis or meconium aspiration syndrome [MAS] with 'ball valve effect') or in healthy newborns breathing their first breaths, underventilated areas allow the overdistention of ventilated alveoli when high ventilation pressures or long in-

Table 1: Reported Frequencies of Pneumothorax

Normal term infants	0.5%–2%
TTN	5%–10%
HMD	up to 20%
HMD and CPAP	up to 20%
HMD and mechanical ventilation	20%–50%
Meconium aspiration syndrome	up to 50%

TTN = Transient tachypnea of the newborn
CPAP = Continuous positive air pressure

spiratory times are used. The alveoli tethered by adjacent bronchi and blood vessels are less free to expand in all directions and are the most likely to rupture into the adjacent, perivascular loose connective tissue.

Loculated air at this stage produces PIE. The perivascular connective tissue in the extreme premature is more abundant and less dissectable. Air frequently remains trapped at this site, finding its way into the lymphatics. In the mature infant, air usually dissects along this connective tissue plane toward the mediastinum, creating a pneumomediastinum or, with rupture into the pleural space, a pneumothorax. Although the air present in a pneumomediastinum is seldom under tension, very high pleural pressure can result from a pneumothorax. This high pressure may decrease the gradient to blood flow to the right atrium (whose pressure reflects pleural pressure) or cause mediastinal compression. This may then decrease venous return and cardiac output. Occasionally, air dissects from the mediastinum up into subcutaneous tissues of the neck (*subcutaneous emphysema*) or into the abdomen (*pneumoperitoneum*).

Mechanical ventilation increases the risk of air block, especially with ventilatory strategies that favor maldistributed ventilation. Long inspiratory times compromise exhalation times and may cause air trapping. In addition, slower rates require higher tidal volumes to achieve normal minute ventilation, and with abnormal distribution of ventilation, overdistention can occur. Hand bagging, especially by the inexperienced, may result in high pressures and long inspiratory times. Bronchial intubation may create overexpansion of the ventilated lung and atelectasis of the contralateral lung, especially with volume ventilators. Finally, agitated babies, who cry and fight the ventilator, may have unexpected patterns of ventilation resulting in alveolar overdistention.

Presentation

History and physical examination. While some pneumothoraces are asymptomatic, the presentation may be precipitous with an acute onset of hypoxemia and even cardiovascular collapse. If symptomatic, a rapid increase in respiratory rate and symptoms of respiratory distress are virtually always found. An increasing anterioposterior diameter on the affected side is a dependable sign, although uncommon. Decreased breath sounds and chest excursion, while suggestive, are nonspecific. Heart sounds may become muffled, and the point of maximum impulse may shift. If venous return is obstructed, diastolic blood pressure may be increased and cardiac output decreased. If cardiac output is affected, tachycardia, bradycardia, or evidence of systolic hypotension and decreased pulses may be found.

Even with large collections of air, a pneumomediastinum is usually asymptomatic or only associated with mild tachypnea. In some babies, heart sounds may be muffled. Subcutaneous emphysema is recognized by the palpable crepitant mass in the neck, upper thorax, or scalp. The clinical manifestations of a pneumoperitoneum vary with the volume of air and the presence or absence of tension. Many are asymptomatic. If there is sufficient tension, the functional residual capacity of the lung may be compromised and venous return to the heart may decrease secondary to compression of the inferior vena cava.

Symptoms of PIE are more insidious than those of a pneumothorax; frequently, onset is first noted on chest radiograph. PIE is primarily manifest by an increasingly noncompliant lung and worsening oxygenation. With sufficient overdistention, venous return and cardiac output are diminished.

Transillumination. A strong, presumptive diagnosis of a pneumothorax can be made without radiograph to avoid postponing treatment in an emergency. Transillumination with a high-intensity, fiberoptic probe in a darkened room has been shown to have high sensitivity and specificity. False negatives may be caused by large infants with increased skin thickness, small collections of air, or situations where the thymus is elevated against the chest wall. False positives are seen with subcutaneous edema, pneumomediastinum, lobar emphysema, or PIE. The transilluminator is applied directly to the skin of the chest wall and gradually moved over alternate sides of the chest. Normally, the ring of light surrounding the probe will extend about 1 cm. A larger or asymmetric ring of light suggests a pneumothorax. When large, the entire chest may light up. Transillumination is less helpful with PIE.

X-ray. If large, a pneumothorax can be easily identified by chest radiograph. Identification of smaller collections can be difficult. Air may be visible only in scattered areas or only along the medial or basilar aspect of the lung. Anterior air may present as a large, hyperlucent hemithorax with increased sharpness at the edge of the mediastinum. A cross-table lateral or a decubitus radiograph can help when doubt exists.

The appearance of a pneumomediastinum can take on a wide variety of configurations, some of which can be quite bizarre. Most typically, air collects around the heart, elevating the lobes of the thymus. This can resemble a billowing spinnaker sail of a racing yacht, hence this finding is referred

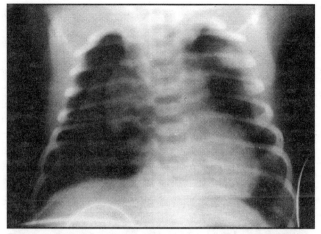

Figure 1: Pneumomediastinum and right-sided pneumothorax. This radiograph shows the right lobe of the thymus as lifted up and away from the cardiac silhouette in the typical 'spinnaker sail' configuration. The left lobe of the thymus also appears in the superior left hemithorax and might be confused with a mass or area of consolidation. A moderately large pneumothorax is seen on the right as a dark area without pulmonary parenchymal markings.

to as the 'spinnaker sail' sign. When both lobes of the thymus are elevated, an 'angel wing' configuration has been described. When a large volume of mediastinal air is present, the thymic lobes can be elevated far into the apex of the chest and can be mistaken for atelectasis or an intrapulmonary mass.

Differentiation of a pneumomediastinum from a medial pneumothorax can be challenging. Medial pneumothoraces, which normally lie lateral to the lobes of the thymus, are usually observed when the volume is small to moderate (Figure 1). Differentiation can be aided by a lateral view. With a pneumomediastinum, an area of extreme hyperlucency in the *superior* retrosternal space is almost always seen. An

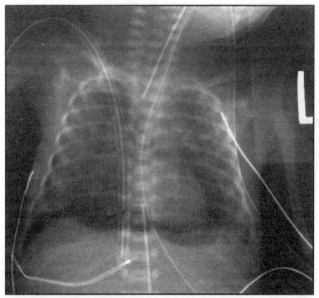

Figure 2: Pneumopericardium. This infant, who has previously had a right pneumothorax, now presents with an air-filled pericardial sac. This is distinguishable from a pneumomediastinum or medial pneumothorax by the air found beneath the cardiac silhouette and the outline of the pericardial sac.

anterior pneumothorax more often occupies the entire superior surface of the heart. Rarely, air from a pneumomediastinum may lie below the heart and may be confused with a pneumopericardium. Generally, air from a pneumopericardium not only lies below, but also totally encircles the heart (Figure 2).

In infants with PIE, the chest radiograph (Figure 3) is most remarkable for tortuous 2- to 3-mm-diameter bubbles of air that follow the perivascular sheaths from the hilum and do not empty with expiratory films. With progression of the PIE (and often over just a few hours), the bubbles become less tortuous and develop into larger cysts. As a result of the air

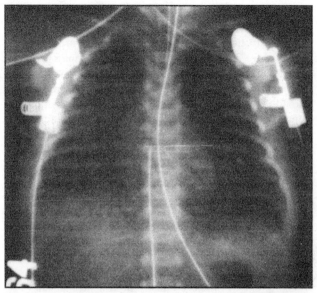

Figure 3: Pulmonary interstitial emphysema (PIE). In this premature infant, the bubbly changes are seen throughout both lungs. In many infants, they are more prominent toward the hilum and may appear to be air bronchograms. The bubbles in PIE are larger and less uniform in outline than those seen in hyaline membrane disease. The lungs have a large volume, flattening the diaphragm and squeezing the heart (which is only about 40% of the thoracic diameter).

trapping, the lung volume is large and depression of the diaphragm can become profound. Decreased venous return and hypoxic vasoconstriction may result in a general darkening of the lung fields. PIE is frequently associated with other forms of extrapleural air (eg, pneumothorax or pneumopericardium).

Laboratory. Pneumothoraces and PIE will both be manifested by decreased blood oxygen levels and carbon dioxide retention. There may be a mixed respiratory and metabolic acidosis.

Management of Pneumothorax

A small-volume, asymptomatic pneumothorax may only require observation. Although a nitrogen washout in a 100% oxygen hood for 24 to 48 hours has been used to manage mildly symptomatic, term infants, there are significant potential morbidities that should be considered, and unmonitored oxygen should not be used. The risk of administering high oxygen concentrations for a disease with such little morbidity seems excessive. Nitrogen washout can only occur in the total absence of nitrogen (see *Ventilation-Perfusion Relationships* section, Chapter 2). Consequently, less than 100% oxygen will not wash out nitrogen.

In an emergency, air may be aspirated with a 22- to 25-g scalp vein needle placed over the superior aspect of the rib in the midclavicular line. The clinician should place the end in a sterile water bottle or apply a syringe and aspirate just enough to relieve symptoms. This should avoid damage to the lung and allow for subsequent chest-tube placement.

Symptomatic infants or those requiring mechanical ventilation most likely will require chest tube placement. The goal is to place the tip of the chest tube between the lung and the anterior chest wall. After appropriate analgesia and sterile preparation, incise the skin at the first to third intercostal space at the midclavicular line or the sixth to seventh intercostal space at the midaxillary line. Avoid the tissue of the areola or breast. Then bluntly dissect with a curved hemostat. Tunnel one to two interspaces to the second intercostal space at the midclavicular line or the fourth or fifth space at the midaxillary line. Insert an 8- to 12-F chest tube without trocar. Direct the tube anteriorly to optimize drainage of air and connect to 10- to 15-cm H_2O continuous suction. Secure with a suture and cover with antibiotic ointment and an occlusive dressing. A chest radiograph will verify placement and effectiveness. A lateral radiograph helps determine anterior-vs-posterior positioning. Complications of chest tube insertion include inadvertent placement in the subcutaneous tissue, as well as perforations of the pulmonary parenchyma that occur up to 35% of the time and usually heal uneventfully without developing a bronchopleural fistula. Chest tubes may bruise the diaphragm or mediastinal structures, producing paralysis or erosion.

Generally, the air leak will resolve after several days. Continued bubbling suggests that a hole of the chest tube may be lying outside the chest, loose connections in the drainage equipment, air leak at the incision site, or a pleural fistula. Consider removal of the tube when there has been no bubbling for 24 hours, and no air is seen on the chest radiograph. Before removal of the tube, place the tube to underwater seal for 24 hours, clamp the tube for a time, then remove rapidly. Apply an occlusive dressing to the wound. Follow up with chest radiograph and observe for recurrence.

Pneumomediastinum. Mediastinal air seldom achieves sufficient pressure to compromise circulation, and specific treatment is not required. Clinical observation is important because these babies can deteriorate if a pneumothorax develops.

PIE. The keys to successful management of PIE are early recognition, minimization of further air leak, and adjustment of ventilatory goals. Serial chest radiographs and a high index of suspicion in infants at risk for PIE are critical.

PIE produces extrinsic pressure on airways leading to adjacent alveoli and can result in gas trapping in these units. Interruption of this cycle is achieved by maneuvers that decrease ventilation to these poorly ventilated areas. Because of increased airway resistance, the time constant (see *Lung Mechanics,* Chapter 2) to these areas is longer than in the normally ventilated unit. Shortening the inspiratory time to 0.1 to 0.15 seconds will selectively decrease ventilation to the PIE-affected alveoli. Compensation with higher peak inspiratory pressures (PIP) may then be required to maintain oxygenation and ventilation. Minimize these changes and provide positive end expiratory pressure (PEEP) just sufficient to prevent airway collapse. Both higher PIP and PEEP *exacerbate* air trapping.

To avoid excessive ventilation settings, the clinician may need to modify the desired Pao_2, $Paco_2$, and pH. Accept Pao_2 of 35 to 45 while minimizing oxygen consumption, optimizing hemoglobin and circulatory status, and monitoring for worsening lactic acidosis. Elevations in the $Paco_2$ are acceptable, as long as the pH remains greater than 7.15 to 7.20. Occasionally, PIE will be unilateral; it then may be helpful to selectively intubate the less affected side or position the baby with that side up. Some institutions have had success using high-frequency ventilation (see *High-Frequency Jet Ventilation* and *High-Frequency Oscillatory Ventilation* sections, Chapter 10).

Pneumopericardium. In the presence of life-threatening tamponade, a pericardial drain can be inserted using the following steps: the clinician should prepare an 18- to 20-gauge IV cannula by attaching an IV extension tube, open stopcock, and syringe. Cover the transilluminator tip with a sterile glove to allow use within the sterile field. After appropriate analgesia and skin preparation, the clinician should make a small stab wound in the left xiphosternal angle and insert the IV cannula, directing it toward the tip of the left scapula, using the transilluminator as a guide to outline the pneumopericardium. Applying constant suction on the syringe, the cannula is advanced until air is evacuated. If the air reaccumulates, the cannula should be secured, placed to continuous suction, and its position confirmed by chest radiograph. Frequently, the small internal diameter of the IV cannula does not provide sufficient drainage. In this case, consider a more permanent tube placed by cutdown.

Outcome

While most infants with pneumothoraces will have an uneventful recovery, they may have a higher mortality and morbidity. In our very-low-birth-weight infants, mortality increased by threefold to fourfold with air block. Air embolization is rare but fatal when it occurs. Pleural fistulas may require open thoracotomy. Subsequent bronchopulmonary dysplasia (BPD) appears to be more frequent. The incidence of intraventricular hemorrhage increases. This may be associated with impaired venous return and hypercarbia-induced increase in cerebral blood flow or, alternatively, from sudden improvement in cerebral perfusion after chest tube placement. Symptoms of inappropriate antidiuresis hormone (SIADH) have been reported.

Infants with PIE have a much more guarded prognosis. They have a higher incidence of pneumopericardium. Their mortality is significantly higher, as is their incidence of subsequent BPD; it may be as high as 50%.

By Timothy R. Cooper, MD

Chronic Pulmonary Insufficiency of Prematurity

Chronic pulmonary insufficiency of prematurity (CPIP), or late onset respiratory distress, is less a disease than the physiologic consequences of prematurity. As described in Chapter 2, resting lung volume is determined by the balance of forces favoring collapse (spontaneous atelectasis of the lung) and the forces favoring expansion (the spring outwards of the chest wall). The extreme premature weighing less than 1,200 g has a soft, flexible chest wall, with poorly ossified ribs and diminished muscle mass. In addition, the predominant sleep activity is rapid eye movement (REM), a time when tonic intercostal muscle activity is diminished and phasic activity is curtailed. Furthermore, the ribs lie more nearly horizontal, further decreasing the efficiency of the accessory respiratory muscles.

Finally, the flatter configuration and narrower zone of apposition of the diaphragm make *this* organ of respiration less effective as well. All these forces taken together favor alveolar collapse.

CPIP is characterized by the development of apnea, respiratory difficulty, and increasing oxygen requirements during the first weeks of life. Blood gases and pulmonary function testing show modest hypercapnia and an increased transalveolar gradient for O_2, CO_2, and N_2 (increased $AaDo_2$, $aADco_2$, and $aADn_2$). Poorly defined, diffuse hazy-appearing parenchyma are seen on the chest radiograph.

We find a very good response to nasal continuous positive airway pressure (N-CPAP) administered until the baby is greater than 1,200 to 1,300 g or about 30 weeks' gestation. Caffeine helps by decreasing apnea, decreasing REM sleep, and increasing diaphragmatic and accessory muscle tone. If on weaning or discontinuing N-CPAP, the baby has an increase in oxygen requirement or apnea, then the baby should be returned to the previous level of support. This suggests a loss of lung volume resulting in hypoventilation and an elevated alveolar Pco_2 and hence lower alveolar Po_2. These signs may take 24 to 48 hours to develop as the infant gradually loses lung volume. Because continued growth will improve chest wall stability, the weaning attempts may be periodically repeated until successful.

By Timothy R. Cooper, MD

Bronchopulmonary Dysplasia

Bronchopulmonary dysplasia (BPD) is the clinical evolution of a sequence of injuries beginning with the initial interface of mechanical ventilation and the lung of the vulnerable host. This process progresses either to death or to recovery after 1 to 3 years of lung growth.

Occurrence is inversely related to birth weight, exceeding 75% in those below 751 g birth weight. The classic definition of bronchopulmonary dysplasia has been a continued need for oxygen beyond 28 days of life. It has been suggested, however, that the definition be narrowed to those infants requiring oxygen supplementation or mechanical ventilation beyond 36 weeks' gestation. Because risk of death and major morbidity are closely related to chronic ventilator course, management of the ventilator-dependent infant is the focus of this section.

Etiology and Pathogenesis

Suggested etiologies have included pulmonary immaturity, oxygen toxicity, barotrauma, volutrauma, vitamin deficiency, failed antioxidant protection, excess fluid administration, patent ductus arteriosus (PDA), and chronic infection (eg, from *Ureaplasma*, *Chlamydia*, or cytomegalovirus). Although oxidant injury remains an important area of investigation, recent work has led to a comprehensive concept of a lung injury sequence that evolves after activation of inflammatory mediators by acute ventilator-induced injury. In survivors, this is followed by a prolonged and disordered process of repair and resolution. This view emphasizes the primary importance of airway injury in the clinical course of BPD.

Genetic predisposition is suggested by an increased family history of asthma among BPD patients, as well as by evidence of early airway injury in certain very-low-birth-weight subgroups. Goldman demonstrated that mean pulmonary resistance among ventilated prematures in the first 5 days of life was about 90% higher in those subsequently developing BPD. The surfactant-deficient or structurally immature lung is particularly vulnerable to bronchiolar lesions induced by mechanical ventilation and disruption of airways that occurs very early in the course of mechanical ventilation.

A unifying concept that explains induction of this airway injury is that of 'volutrauma.' Relative risk of BPD increases with decreasing P_{CO_2} below 40 mm Hg, an effect particularly striking with P_{CO_2} values below 29 mm Hg. Experimentally, if the chest is bound to prevent lung expansion, transpulmonary pressures above 50 cm H_2O may be applied without air leak or lung injury. Pulmonary edema induced by high tidal volume ventilation can also be prevented by chest binding. Such data suggest that acute lung injury is determined by the relationship between delivered maximum lung volume (V_{max}) and tidal volume. As tidal volume approaches the V_{max} of an individual lung, airways become overdistended and geometrically distorted. Thus, volume-induced injury may occur in immature lungs with a low V_{max} even at low ventilator pressures, because the delivered tidal volume plus any positive end-expiratory pressure (PEEP) applied may be near the V_{max} for those lungs. Shearing and disruption are associated with necrosis of bronchial mucosa and activation of an intense inflammatory response, leading to further lung damage and progressive clinical symptoms.

Clinical Course

The clinical course of BPD in the surfactant era is more insidious than originally described by Northway (Table 2). Most patients are surfactant-treated infants, <1,250 g at birth, without hyaline membrane disease, but requiring mechanical ventilation during the first week of life because of apnea or structural immaturity of the lungs. The course of the chronically ventilator-dependent infant can be divided into three clinical phases.

Phase I—Acute course and diagnosis. This evolves during the first month of life and most closely corresponds to Northway stages 1 and 2. A relatively benign course during the first 2 weeks gives way to continued ventilator dependency with progressive deterioration in pulmonary function, rising oxygen requirements, and opacification of previously clear lung fields on chest radiograph. Wide swings in Po_2 and oxygen saturation values are characteristic. Despite treatment of PDA, effective use of xanthines for apnea, and lack of evidence of infection, the infant remains ventilator dependent. Marked increases in microvascular permeability occur, and there is widespread necrosis of bronchial mucosa. Numerous inflammatory markers are found in tracheal fluid of these babies compared with those with no signs of chronic pulmonary disease. Airways are obstructed with necrotic debris, and atelectasis may alternate with early cyst formation. Within 3 to 4 weeks, a process of exclusion has established BPD as the cause of persistent ventilator dependency.

Table 2: Northway's Stages of Bronchopulmonary Dysplasia

Stage	Chest Radiograph Findings
1.	Consistent with HMD.
2.	Opaque lung fields with air bronchograms. Interstitial air is common.
3.	Cystic lung fields with areas of hyperinflation and areas of atelectasis.
4.	Massive lung fibrosis and edema; areas of consolidation and areas of overinflation.

Phase II—Course of chronic ventilator dependency. This phase includes features of Northway stages 3 and 4. Bronchiolar metaplasia, hypertrophy of smooth muscle, and interstitial edema produce uneven airway obstruction with worsening hyperinflation of the lung. Obliteration and abnormal muscularization of the pulmonary vascular bed progresses. Active inflammation slowly subsides to be replaced by a disordered process of structural repair. The early weeks of this phase remain quite unstable with frequent changes in oxygen requirement and characteristic episodes of acute deterioration, requiring increases in ventilator support. After 4 to 6 weeks, the clinical course becomes more static as fibrosis, hyperinflation, and pulmonary edema come to dominate the clinical picture. Increased airway smooth muscle is present, and tracheobronchomalacia is common. Chronic elevation of pulmonary vascular resistance (PVR) increases right ventricular afterload, impairs pulmonary lymphatic drainage, and leaves the infant vulnerable to episodes of acute cor pulmonale.

The course of phase II evolves over 3 to 9 months. During this time, growth and remodeling of both the lung parenchyma and the pulmonary vascular bed are associated with gradual improvement in pulmonary function and heart-lung interaction. Oxygen requirements fall to 40% or less, and the patient can be weaned from intermittent positive pressure ventilation (IPPV) to breathe spontaneously on continuous positive airway pressure (CPAP) or a pressure support mode of ventilation. Subsequently, extubation and supplemental oxygen alone become sufficient.

Phase III—Discharge planning and transition to home care. This phase covers the transition from mechanical ventilation to the home care environment. Active, inflammatory lung damage has ceased, and the process of repair has become more orderly. Lung growth and remodeling of parenchyma and vasculature have progressed sufficiently to allow more stable pulmonary function without the need for positive pressure support. Lung mechanics, especially airway resistance, remain quite abnormal, however, and hyperinflation, fibrosis, and cysts often remain visible radiographically. Many more months of lung growth will be required to overcome these derangements.

The most important aspect of this phase is the recognition that, although the lung has improved, both structure and function remain abnormal. Close monitoring of adequacy of oxygenation is essential for several weeks after extubation to be sure a subtle rise in PVR will not lead to insidious development of cor pulmonale. During this period, discharge planning can begin. Hearing and developmental screening can proceed, along with increased attention to play therapy and any required physical therapy. Many infants will have problems with oral motor function and feeding. Effects of feeding on oxygenation must be evaluated closely. Special home care needs should be identified, and a home dietary plan chosen and implemented. Most of these infants will be discharged with low flow oxygen by nasal cannula, an oral diuretic, and modest fluid restriction (150 mL/kg/d) using a standard 24 kcal/oz formula that is readily available commercially. Continuation of nebulized albuterol by mask is often necessary. As long as the infant requires oxygen, both fluid restriction and diuretics will make lung function more efficient and help minimize PVR.

Cardiopulmonary Physiology

In advanced BPD, there is a marked increase in airway resistance and a decrease in dynamic compliance, which becomes frequency dependent. Tidal volume is reduced and respiratory rate is increased. The uneven airway obstruction leads to gas trapping and hyperinflation with severe pulmonary clearance delay. Only 36% of the functional residual capacity (FRC) is composed of well-ventilated lung units. If bronchomalacia is present, forced airway collapse may occur during active expiratory efforts associated with agitation. Little improvement in pulmonary function occurs before 6 months of age. By 3 years of age, compliance is near normal, and airway resistance is only about 30% higher than controls.

The fragile heart-lung interaction in these patients can be depicted as a three-compartment model. In one compartment, airways, gas exchange units, and blood vessels have been obliterated, producing a reduction in cross-sectional area of the pulmonary vascular bed and gas exchange surface. In the second compartment, uneven airway obstruction produces a population of underventilated (though often hyperinflated) lung units in which alveolar hypoxia induces hypoxic pulmonary vasoconstriction. This adds to a further increase in resting PVR. The third compartment, with well-ventilated lung units and intact vasculature, must accept a disproportionate amount of pulmonary blood flow. These vessels, already maximally dilated, can only accept additional flow at the expense of high right ventricular afterload, high microvascular pressures, and increased fluid filtration into the perivascular interstitium. Chronically elevated right-sided cardiac pressures also inhibit pulmonary lymphatic drainage. Any further reduction in ventilation or fall in P_{AO_2} in the underventilated compartment (such as that accompanying mucous plugging, bronchospasm, or reduction in F_{IO_2}) induces additional regional hypoxic vasoconstriction and forces yet more blood through the well-ventilated compartment, with further increase in pulmonary edema.

Understanding this fragile heart-lung interaction is the essence of management of BPD. Pulmonary care is designed to minimize PVR, especially in the underventilated compartment, so to avoid the vicious circle of pulmonary edema causing deterioration in pulmonary function, which in turn causes more pulmonary edema, a course eventually terminating in acute right ventricular failure.

Management

Primary goals of management.

- Provision of complete, balanced nutrition together with time, to allow growth of new lung and remodeling of the pulmonary vascular bed;
- Avoidance of cor pulmonale, a major cause of death, by providing comprehensive care and monitoring to minimize PVR.

Recovery of the ventilator-dependent infant will occur only over months. During this period, care is largely supportive and primarily improves short-term oxygenation and reduces work of breathing, without changing the underlying repair process. Attempting to wean supplemental oxygen too quickly risks increases in PVR, which may precipitate acute cardiopulmonary failure.

Supportive care and nutrition. Growth and development of new airways, gas exchange units, and pulmonary vasculature require 1 to 3 years and the provision of all primary and trace nutrients. A balanced nutrient intake must be provided in conjunction with fluid restriction, increased mineral wasting from diuretic therapy, and, at times, the catabolic effects of corticosteroids. Long-term dietary intake should meet all guidelines of the American Academy of Pediatrics for term and preterm infants.

Infants with BPD benefit from fluid restriction to control pulmonary edema. In preterm infants, modest fluid restriction (150 mL/kg/d) is compatible with proper long-term nutrition using one of the commercial 24 kcal/oz, mineral-enhanced premature formulas. These provide good quality protein intake, trace nutrients, and increased calcium and phosphorus supplementation to optimize bone mineralization. When the infant reaches term, a standard 24 kcal/oz formula may be substituted. If necessary, additional calories may be added as corn oil. At this level of fluid restriction, adequate growth may be possible using human milk with added commercial fortifier containing supplemental protein, minerals, and vitamins. Such infants require close monitoring of growth and bone mineral status.

Severe impairment of lung mechanics may require restriction of fluids to 110 to 120 mL/kg/d. Adding caloric supplements alone to a 24 kcal/oz formula will not support growth at this low intake. Protein and trace nutrients will be deficient. A commercial 27 kcal/oz formula may be fortified with protein (eg, Casec®) to achieve an intake of 3 to 3.5 g/kg/d of protein. Addition of corn oil and glucose polymers can increase caloric density to 30 to 32 kcal/oz. Such mixtures, however, will exceed an osmolarity of 410 mOsm/L. In babies more than 5 to 6 months of age, adequate nutrition can be maintained using 100 to 120 mL/kg/d of a liquid diet formulated for older infants. Pediasure® with Fiber (Ross Laboratories, Columbus, Ohio) has been shown to produce mean weight gain of 30 g/d in infants with BPD requiring severe fluid restriction. Feedings may be initiated with full-strength Pediasure® at 110 to 120 mL/kg/d. If renal solute load proves excessive, the product may be diluted to three-fourths strength and given at 135 mL/kg/d. Infants receiving a special formula in restricted amounts require iron and vitamin supplements.

Diuretics. Diuretics improve short-term lung mechanics and may promote a reduction in oxygen requirements or ventilator support. Two reported regimens have facilitated improvement in lung function and enhanced weaning from IPPV while minimizing effects of hypochloremic metabolic alkalosis.

(1) Furosemide (1 mg/kg/dose, b.i.d., IV or 2 mg/kg/dose, b.i.d., enterally) given every other day is as effective

as daily dosing and results in much less chloride depletion and urinary calcium loss.

(2) Hydrochlorothiazide (2 mg/kg/dose, b.i.d.) or chlorothiazide (20 mg/kg/dose, b.i.d.) combined with spironolactone (1.5 mg/kg/dose, b.i.d.) may be given daily. This regimen has improved lung mechanics and reduced urinary calcium excretion in some studies, but may be associated with increased potassium and phosphorus loss.

Chronic diuretic therapy usually requires chloride supplementation of 2 to 4 mEq/kg/d above usual nutritional needs. At least one third should be provided as KCl.

Oxygen. Development of pulmonary hypertension is a predictor of mortality in BPD. Oxygen is the primary tool to minimize PVR and avoid death from cor pulmonale. FIO_2 should be adjusted to maintain arterial Pao_2 above 55 mm Hg. Insidious hypoxemia is particularly common during feedings and sleep, when additional oxygen supplements may be necessary. Need for supplemental oxygen extends well beyond the period of positive-pressure support. The impact of oxygen on outcome cannot be overemphasized, because overzealous attempts to wean supplemental oxygen may precipitate acute cardiopulmonary failure and even death.

Bronchodilators. Increased resting airway tone has been demonstrated in infants with BPD, and numerous studies have reported improved lung mechanics after administration of β-agonists to ventilator-dependent infants.

Although a sound basis exists for bronchodilator therapy in BPD, clinical use is largely empiric. Bedside pulmonary function testing in small infants lacks adequate sensitivity to select specific responders to different treatment regimens and to guide the course of daily management. The major drawback to this therapy is the high cumulative cost. In the absence of sensitive bedside pulmonary function testing, the empiric use of routine bronchodilator therapy has a place in the long-term care of most patients.

(1) Albuterol: Denjean described a dose-response relationship for ventilator-dependent prematures using a metered dose inhaler (MDI) to administer 1 or 2 puffs (90 or 180 µg) of albuterol, q 3 h into a commercial spacer device. This device is placed between the ventilator circuit connector and the endotracheal tube connector. For older, larger infants up to 6 puffs per treatment may be required.

(2) Ipratropium bromide: Limited data suggest this agent, at inhaled doses of 25 µg/kg, lowers respiratory system resistance in some preterm infants with BPD in a manner similar to albuterol. A dose-dependent effect has been demonstrated in older children with asthma at doses of 75 to 250 µg per treatment. In asthmatic infants less than 1 year of age, clinical improvement has been reported with this dosage range. No specific side effects were reported in these limited studies. Administration to intubated patients can be accomplished using an MDI and spacer device connected to the endotracheal tube. Although the idea of synergy with β_2-agonists is appealing, a definitive role for cholinergic blockade in these patients has not been established.

(3) Inhaled corticosteroids: No clear role for use of inhaled corticosteroids has been established in BPD, but this route could represent a desirable alternative to systemic therapy, especially in chronic use. LaForce reported improved airway resistance and lung compliance in a group of ventilator-dependent preterm infants after nebulization of beclomethasone for more than 2 weeks (50 µg/2 mL normal saline, nebulized into the ventilator circuit t.i.d.). The incidence of infection was not increased in the small

group studied. Alternatively, this drug may be given by MDI using a commercial spacer device connected to the endotracheal tube.

Acute episodes of bronchospasm do occur in some infants with BPD. For severe episodes of airway reactivity, albuterol is the agent of choice. It may be given by MDI and spacer or by nebulization (0.15 mg/kg in 2.0 mL NS) into the ventilator circuit every 20 minutes for 1 to 2 hours. A minimum dose of 1.25 mg is recommended for infants by the National Institutes of Health (NIH) Asthma Panel Guidelines. If there is no response, continuous nebulization of 0.5 mg/kg/h may be given for 1 to 2 hours. Note, however, that nebulization into ventilator circuits has been associated with wide variations in dose delivery, rainout of fluid, cooling of inspired gas, and significant changes in airway pressures.

Systemic corticosteroids. Initial animal research suggested that corticosteroids might enhance oxygen toxicity, interfere with lung growth, and accelerate pulmonary fibrosis. Subsequent studies, however, have established an increasingly important role for these agents in management of BPD. Three strategies for clinical use have emerged. Numerous controlled trials have demonstrated a reduction in duration of assisted ventilation among infants with established BPD treated with corticosteroids. In this setting, short-term lung mechanics are improved, in part by a brisk diuresis and decrease in lung water. Adrenal suppression can be avoided if the course of treatment does not exceed 1 week. To optimize response to a pulse course of treatment, the patient should be receiving adequate ventilator support, oxygen, fluid restriction (150 mL/kg/d or less), and an effective regimen of diuretics. Dexamethasone can be given by many regimens. One is to begin with 0.25 mg/kg/d, b.i.d. for 48 to 72 hours, then tapered by 50% per day over the next 3 to 5 days. This allows for completion of therapy after 1 week. Because response occurs early in the course of corticosteroid therapy, babies failing to wean from IPPV after 1 week of treatment are unlikely to do so subsequently. Some infants who initially respond, however, require continued corticosteroid therapy.

More recent studies have focused on early treatment to interrupt the lung injury cycle. Dexamethasone given during the first 2 weeks of life has been reported to reduce oxygen requirements, reduce duration of ventilator support, and decrease need for supplemental oxygen at 36 weeks' postmenstrual age. Many of these infants, however, required either repeated courses of treatment or continued daily therapy for as long as 42 days. Reported side effects were hypertension and glucose intolerance.

A preventive role for corticosteroid therapy is also being investigated. Recent reports suggest dexamethasone (0.5 mg to 1.0 mg/kg/d) initiated in the first 12 hours of postnatal life results in earlier extubation and less oxygen dependency at 36 weeks' postmenstrual age. Effects were particularly notable in surfactant-treated prematures of <1,250 g at birth. Study design for duration of treatment in these reports varied between 1 and 12 days. Hypertension and glucose intolerance were again common side effects. Incidence of infection was not increased in treated infants, but growth failure was reported.

The risks of long-term corticosteroid therapy compared with chronic ventilation in small prematures must be weighed carefully. Several early studies reported increased rates of infection, but the incidence of sepsis has not been increased in most reports involving early treatment and short courses of therapy. Hypertension, though common, rarely requires specific intervention. Suppression of growth and adrenal function, however, remain potentially serious clinical problems.

Preventive care. Attempts to prevent or ameliorate severity of BPD with administration of antioxidants such as vitamin E and superoxide dismutase have thus far been ineffective. Although premature infants with BPD have been found to have lower serum vitamin A concentrations than others with respiratory distress syndrome (RDS), clinical tri-

161

als involving supplementation have yielded equivocal results. Strategies designed to prevent BPD or to ameliorate severity with early corticosteroid therapy are noted above.

Association of early hypocarbia and subsequent BPD has strengthened the concept of volutrauma and fostered several strategies for gentle ventilation. These combine low pressures, low tidal volumes, and short inspiratory times with permissive hypercarbia. Early use of nasal CPAP represents an attempt to avoid ventilator-induced injury altogether. A reduction in barotrauma or volume-induced lung injury has been cited in select clinical trials of high-frequency oscillatory ventilation reporting a reduced incidence of BPD.

Infection, particularly respiratory syncytial virus (RSV), is a significant cause of postdischarge hospitalization and death in these patients. Recent trials suggest RSV intravenous immune globulin (RespiGam™) reduces incidence and total days of hospitalization among infants younger than 24 months with BPD. The American Academy of Pediatrics currently recommends that infants with BPD who are receiving oxygen or have received it within the 6 months before the RSV season be considered for RespiGam™ prophylaxis. A monthly infusion of 750 mg/kg/dose is recommended, beginning before the onset of RSV season and repeated monthly until its seasonal termination. Intravenous administration of this product presents significant logistical problems, however, and requires a fluid load of 15 mL/kg/dose (see *Discharge Planning,* Chapter 13). Clinical trials of an alternative intramuscular product are underway.

Monitoring of Course and Coordination of Care

A comprehensive program of monitoring is necessary to achieve adequate growth and avoid cor pulmonale.

Nutritional monitoring. Patients should be weighed every 1 to 3 days and length and frontal-occipital circumference measurements should be obtained weekly. Nutritional monitoring should include periodic determination of blood urea nitrogen (BUN), serum albumin, prealbumin, calcium, phosphorus, and alkaline phosphatase. A dietitian or physician with special skills in infant nutrition should be a member of the care team and periodically evaluate dietary profile and growth parameters.

Oxygen monitoring. Long-term maintenance of adequate oxygenation is the key to preventing death from cor pulmonale. Adequacy of oxygenation can be evaluated by obtaining a 6- to 8-hour strip recording of transcutaneous oxygen tension ($TcPo_2$) or pulse oximetry (Spo_2) every 1 to 2 weeks. Attempts should be made to keep $TcPo_2$ above 55 mm Hg and Spo_2 above 94% in term and older infants (90% to 95% range in small prematures). Arterial blood gas samples must be obtained periodically, but may be difficult to interpret because of agitation or sampling difficulties.

Echocardiograms. The value of echocardiography in screening for pulmonary hypertension and assessing response of the pulmonary vascular bed to oxygen has been described in several studies. Tricuspid regurgitation is common, and flow velocity can be determined by Doppler. A modified Bernoulli equation can be used to calculate the pressure gradient across this valve [pressure gradient = $4(V_{max})^2$]. This value plus assumed right atrial pressure provides an estimate of right ventricular systolic pressure. Increased mortality risk has been associated with PEP/RVET ratios >0.30 and it is recommended that sufficient oxygen be given to avoid ratios >0.34. These two echocardiographic parameters can be measured every 4 to 6 weeks to estimate right ventricular afterload and assess adequacy of pulmonary care. If either is abnormal, an increase in supplemental oxygen, as well as other components of pulmonary care, should be considered.

Developmental screening. Hearing screening should be done prior to discharge or before 6 months of age to allow early intervention by an audiologist, if needed. Developmental assessment may begin during the hospital stay as part of comprehensive long-term follow-up after discharge. Specific attention to oral motor dysfunction and feeding disorders may be necessary.

Planned, multidisciplinary care. Primary goals of care can best be achieved by a multidisciplinary care team directed by an experienced neonatologist or pediatric pulmonologist complemented by other physicians skilled in developmental assessment and nutrition. Team members include nurses, social workers, respiratory therapists, child life specialists, physical and occupational therapists, a dietitian, and an audiologist. The team should have regularly scheduled meetings and rounds to evaluate progress of each patient in regard to goals of care. Such a team can maintain consistent, goal-directed care for each patient with a long-term view. The team is particularly adept at establishing a social environment that minimizes adverse aspects of chronic ventilator care and the ICU environment. Early in the course of ventilator dependency, prematures can benefit from environmental modifications that reduce noise and discomfort and minimize the stress response. As infants become older, parents and caregivers must work together to provide a friendly, play-oriented environment. Some infants with BPD have associated neurologic dysfunction or hearing deficits. Feeding disorders are common. Resources to manage such disorders must be assembled and integrated into a regular schedule of play therapy against a backdrop of ongoing medical care. Maintenance of an appropriate social environment for these chronically hospitalized infants presents a considerable challenge and has significant impact on the medical course. Because prognosis for long-term recovery in BPD is good, the psychology of BPD care is particularly important. It is essential that caregivers maintain an involved, optimistic attitude toward these infants.

Outcome

Outcome varies widely among different centers, with overall mortality ranging from 25% to 40%. Survival to discharge is strongly related to duration of ventilation. Death rates of 21% to 57% are reported for infants requiring more than 1 month of IPPV and may reach 90% when ventilation exceeds 4 months. Most deaths are related to infection or cardiopulmonary failure associated with persistent pulmonary hypertension and cor pulmonale. Improvement in pulmonary function occurs slowly over 1 to 3 years.

Significant increases in growth failure, hearing loss, retinopathy of prematurity (ROP), and neurodevelopmental handicaps have been reported. However, Sauve found only a slight increase in the rate of hearing and developmental abnormalities in a population compared to matched controls, although growth failure and ROP occurred with increased frequency. In an 8-year follow-up study by Robertson, growth of BPD patients born <32 weeks' gestation was similar to that of matched controls. Multivariate analysis suggested that developmental disabilities found among groups of BPD patients were primarily related to complications of prematurity and adverse social factors.

By James M. Adams, MD, and Mary E. Wearden, MD

Wilson-Mikity Syndrome
Epidemiology
Only rarely described since the use of CPAP, this syndrome was said to affect premature infants weighing less than 1,500 g. Although the etiology is unknown, males appear to be affected more often.

Pathophysiology
Although autopsy changes have rarely been reported, they include cystic emphysematous areas interspersed with areas of collapse, cellular thickening of the alveolar septa, increase in fibroelastic tissue, and patchy emphysema. Hypersecretion, aspiration, or immature structure may result in localized pulmonary collapse and air trapping, decreased lung compliance, and increased airway resistance. Higher mean airway pressure from CPAP may prevent this process.

Presentation

Infants with no history of respiratory distress, symptoms of tachypnea, cyanosis, hypercapnia, retractions, or apnea develop this disease between 1 and 4 weeks of age. These symptoms may progress for about 2 months. The infants usually become oxygen dependent, with slow recovery and resolution during the ensuing 1 to 2 years.

The chest radiographic findings are indistinguishable from those of BPD. They progress from the initial coarse, nodular infiltrates, to the development of hyperexpansion, with cystlike changes in the lung. These classic 'bubbly' changes appear to result from areas of alveolar overexpansion surrounded by areas of atelectasis.

Differential Diagnosis

The condition must be distinguished from BPD and other causes of cystic lung disease. In contrast to BPD, the findings of pulmonary hypertension, right ventricular hypertrophy, and pulmonary fibrosis are uncommon.

Management

Wilson-Mikity syndrome should respond well to nasal CPAP.

Outcome

The reported mortality of 30% to 50% from more than two decades ago is difficult to extrapolate to more recent times. It is expected that the outcome should be better than that observed with BPD. There is usually complete radiographic resolution in survivors by 2 years.

By Timothy R. Cooper, MD

Suggested Reading

Air Block

Allen RW, Jung AL, Lester PD: Effectiveness of chest tube evacuation of pneumothorax in neonates. *J Pediatr* 1981;99:629.

Brooks JG, Bustamante SA, Koops BL, et al: Selective bronchial intubation for the treatment of severe localized pulmonary interstitial emphysema in newborn infants. *Pediatrics* 1977;91:648.

Chernick V, Avery ME: Spontaneous alveolar rupture at birth. *Pediatrics* 1963;32:816.

Meadow WL, Cheromcha D: Successful therapy of unilateral pulmonary emphysema: mechanical ventilation with extremely short inspiratory time. *Am J Perinatol* 1985;2:194.

Ogata E, Gregory GA, Kitterman JA, et al: Pneumothorax in respiratory distress syndrome: incidence and effect on vital signs, blood gases and pH. *Pediatrics* 1976;58:177.

Plenat F, Vert P, Didier F, et al: Pulmonary interstitial emphysema. *Clin Perinatol* 1978;5:351.

Reppert SM, Ment LR, Todres ID: The treatment of pneumopericardium in the newborn infant. *J Pediatr* 1977;905:115.

Varano LA, Maisels MJ: Pneumopericardium in the newborn: diagnosis and pathogenesis. *Pediatrics* 1974;53:941.

Bronchopulmonary Dysplasia

Abman SH, Wolfe RR, Accurso FJ, et al: Pulmonary vascular response to oxygen in infants with severe bronchopulmonary dysplasia. *Pediatrics* 1985;75:80-84.

American Academy of Pediatrics, Committee on Infectious Diseases, Committee on Fetus and Newborn. *Pediatrics* 1997;99:645-650.

Avery GB, Fletcher AB, Kaplan M, et al: Controlled trial of dexamethasone in respirator-dependent infants with bronchopulmonary dysplasia. *Pediatrics* 1985;7:106-111.

Bancalari E, et al: Bronchopulmonary dysplasia. *Pediatr Clin North Am* 1996;33:1.

Benatar A, Clarke J, Silverman M: Pulmonary hypertension in infants with chronic lung disease: noninvasive evaluation and short-term effect of oxygen treatment. *Arch Dis Child* 1995;72:F14-F19.

Bolivar JM, Gerhardt T, Gonzalez A, et al: Mechanisms for episodes of hypoxemia in preterm infants undergoing mechanical ventilation. *J Pediatr* 1995;127:767-773.

Brozanski BS, Jones JG, Gilmour CH, et al: Effect of pulse dexamethasone therapy on the incidence and severity of chronic lung disease in the very low birth weight infant. *J Pediatr* 1995;126:769-776.

Carlton DP, Cummings JJ, Scheerer RG, et al: Lung overexpansion increases pulmonary microvascular protein permeability in young lambs. *Am Physiol Soc* 1990;69:577-583.

Collaborative Dexamethasone Trial Group: Dexamethasone therapy in neonatal chronic lung disease: an international placebo-controlled trial. *Pediatrics* 1991;88:421-427.

Committee on Nutrition, American Academy of Pediatrics. *Pediatric Nutrition Handbook.* 3rd ed. Elk Grove, IL: Introduction of Solid Foods (pp 23-32) and Guidelines for Nutrient Intake (pp 64-164).

Davis A, Vickerson F, Worsley G, et al: Determination of dose response relationship for nebulized ipratropium in asthmatic children. *J Pediatr* 1984;105:1002-1005.

Denjean A, Guimaraes H, Migdal M, et al: Dose-related bronchodilator response to aerosolized salbutamol (albuterol) in ventilator-dependent premature infants. *J Pediatr* 1992;120:974-979.

Dryfuss D, Sauman G: Role of tidal volume, FRC and end-expiratory volume in the development of pulmonary edema following mechanical ventilation. *Am Rev Respir Dis* 1993;148:1194-1203.

Durand M, Sardesai S, McEvoy C: Effects of early dexamethasone therapy on pulmonary mechanics and chronic lung disease in very low birth weight infants: a randomized, controlled trial. *Pediatrics* 1995;95:584-590.

Everard ML, Stammers J, Hardy JG, et al: New aerosol delivery system for neonatal ventilator circuits. *Arch Dis Child* 1992;67:826-830.

Fouron J, Le Guennec J, Villemant D, et al: Value of echocardiography in assessing the outcome of bronchopulmonary dysplasia in the newborn. *Pediatrics* 1980;65:529-535.

Garg M, Kruzner SI, Bautista DB, et al: Clinically unsuspected hypoxia during sleep and feeding in infants with bronchopulmonary dysplasia. *Pediatrics* 1988;81:635-642.

Garland JS, Buck RK, Allred EN, et al: Hypocarbia before surfactant therapy appears to increase bronchopulmonary dysplasia risk in infants with respiratory distress syndrome. *Arch Pediatr Adolesc Med* 1995;149:617-623.

Gladstone IM, Jacobs HC, Ehrenkranz RA: Pulmonary function tests and fluid balance in neonates with chronic lung disease during dexamethasone treatment. *Pediatr Res* 1989;25A, Abstract 1277.

Goldman SL, Gerhardt T, Sonni S, et al: Early prediction of chronic lung disease by pulmonary function testing. *J Pediatr* 1983;102:613-616.

Goodman G, Perkin RM, Anas NG, et al: Pulmonary hypertension in infants with bronchopulmonary dysplasia. *J Pediatr* 1988;112:67-72.

Groneck P, Gotze-Speer B, Oppermann M, et al: Association of pulmonary inflammation and increased microvascular permeability during the development of bronchopulmonary dysplasia: a sequential analysis of inflammatory mediators in respiratory fluids of high-risk preterm neonates. *Pediatrics* 1994;93:712-718.

Halliday HL, Dumpit FM, Brady JP: Effects of inspired oxygen on echocardiographic assessments of pulmonary vascular resistance and myocardial contractility in bronchopulmonary dysplasia. *Pediatrics* 1980;65:536-540.

Henry RL, Hiller EJ, Mulner AD, et al: Nebulized ipratropium bromide and sodium cromoglycate in the first two years of life. *Arch Dis Child* 1984;59:54-57.

Hernandez LA, Peevy KJ, Moise AA, et al: Chest wall restriction limits high airway pressure induced lung injury in young rabbits. *Am Physiol Soc* 1989;66(5):2364-2368.

Kao LC, Warburton D, Platzker ACG, et al: Effect of isoproterenol inhalation on airway resistance in chronic bronchopulmonary dysplasia. *Pediatrics* 1984;73:509-513.

Kao LC, Warburton D, Cheng MH: Effect of oral diuretics on pulmonary mechanics in infants with chronic bronchopulmonary dysplasia: results of a double-blind crossover sequential trial. *Pediatrics* 1984;74:37-44.

Kramer R, Birrer P, Modelska K, et al: A new baby spacer device for aerosolized bronchodilator administration in infants with bronchopulmonary disease. *Eur J Pediatr* 1992;151:57-60.

Kraybill EN, Runyan DK, Bose CL, et al: Risk factors for chronic lung disease in infants with birth weights of 751 to 1000 grams. *J Pediatr* 1989;115:115-120.

LaForce WR, Brudno S: Controlled trial of beclomethasone dipropionate by nebulization in oxygen and ventilator dependent infants. *J Pediatr* 1993;122:285-288.

McCubbin M, Frey EE, Wagener JS, et al: Large airway collapse in bronchopulmonary dysplasia. *J Pediatr* 1989;114:304-307.

Miller RW, Woo P, Kellman RK, et al: Tracheobronchial abnormalities in infants with bronchopulmonary dysplasia. *J Pediatr* 1987;111:779-782.

Nilsson R, Grossmann G, Robertson B: Lung surfactant and the pathogenesis of neonatal bronchiolar lesions induced by artificial ventilation. *Pediatr Res* 1978;12:249-255.

Northway WH, Rosan RC, Porter DY: Pulmonary disease following respirator therapy of hyaline membrane disease. *N Engl J Med* 1967;276:357-368.

Overstreet DW, Jackson JC, van Belle G, et al: Estimation of mortality risk in chronically ventilated infants with bronchopulmonary dysplasia. *Pediatrics* 1991;88:1153-1160.

Pearson E, Bose C, Snidlow T, et al: Trial of vitamin A supplementation in very low birth weight infants at risk for bronchopulmonary dysplasia. *J Pediatr* 1992;121:420-427.

Rastogi A, Akintorin SM, Betz ML, et al: A controlled trial of dexamethasone to prevent bronchopulmonary dysplasia in surfactant treated infants. *Pediatrics* 1996;98:204-210.

Robertson B: The evolution of neonatal respiratory distress syndrome into chronic lung disease. *Eur Respir J* 1989;2:33s-37s.

Robertson CMT, Etches PC, Goldson E, et al: Eight-year school performance, neurodevelopmental, and growth outcome of neonates with bronchopulmonary dysplasia: a comparative study. *Pediatrics* 1992;89: 365-372.

Rush MG, Englehardt B, Parker RA, et al: Double-blind, placebo-controlled trial of alternate day furosemide therapy in infants with chronic bronchopulmonary dysplasia. *J Pediatr* 1990;117:112-118.

Sauve RS, Singhal N: Long-term morbidity of infants with bronchopulmonary dysplasia. *Pediatrics* 1985;76:725-733.

Schuh S, Parkin P, Rajan A, et al: High- versus low-dose, frequently administered, nebulized albuterol in children with severe, acute asthma. *Pediatrics* 1989;83:513-518.

Shenai JP, Kennedy KA, Chytil F, et al: Clinical trial of vitamin A supplementation in infants susceptible to bronchopulmonary dysplasia. *J Pediatr* 1987;111:269-277.

Soslulski R, Abbasi S, Fox WW: Therapeutic value of terbutaline in bronchopulmonary dysplasia. *Pediatr Res* 1982;16:309A.

Stephure DK, Singhal N, McMillian DD: Safety of dexamethasone for bronchopulmonary dysplasia. *Pediatr Res* 1989;25, Abstract 546.

U.S. Department of Health and Human Services. *Guidelines for Diagnosis and Management of Asthma.* National Asthma Education Report, Publication No. 91, 3042, 1991.

Valentine C, Schanler R, Abrams S: Appropriate growth of infants 4-12 months of age with bronchopulmonary dysplasia (BPD) using a specialized pediatric formula. *19th Clinical Congress Nutrition Practice* 1995; Poster A177:599.

Watts JL, Ariagno RL, Brady JP: Chronic pulmonary disease in neonates after artificial ventilation: distribution of ventilation and pulmonary interstitial emphysema. *Pediatrics* 1977;60:273-280.

Wheater M, Rennie JM: Poor prognosis after prolonged ventilation for bronchopulmonary dysplasia. *Arch Dis Child* 1994;71:F210-F211.

Wilkie RA, Bryan MH: Effect of bronchodilators on airway resistance in ventilator dependent neonates with chronic lung disease. *J Pediatr* 1987;278-282.

Yeh TF, Torre JA, Rastogi A, et al: Early postnatal dexamethasone therapy in premature infants with severe respiratory distress syndrome: a double-blind, controlled study. *J Pediatr* 1990;117:273-282.

Chronic Pulmonary Insufficiency of Prematurity

Krauss AN, Klain DB, Auld PAM: Chronic pulmonary insufficiency of prematurity (CPIP). *Pediatrics* 1975;55:55.

Wilson-Mikity Syndrome

Burnard ED: The pulmonary syndrome of Wilson and Mikity and respiratory function in very small premature infants. *Pediatr Clin North Am* 1966;13:999.

Hodgman JE, Mikity VG, Tatter D, et al: Chronic respiratory distress in the premature infant. Wilson-Mikity syndrome. *Pediatrics* 1969;44:179.

Krauss AN, Levin AR, Grossman H, et al: Physiologic studies on infants with Wilson-Mikity syndrome. *J Pediatr* 1970;77:27.

Chapter 6

Congenital Diseases Affecting the Lung Parenchyma

Cystic Malformations of the Lung

Cystic malformations are not common causes of respiratory distress. Most are incidental findings in asymptomatic infants. Others present with respiratory distress from recurrent infection, wheezing, or expiratory stridor caused by airway obstruction. On the chest radiograph, round radiolucent cysts may be seen within the pulmonary parenchyma. However, it is often not the cysts per se that draw attention, but the surrounding consolidated or emphysematous parenchyma. With multiple cysts, a diaphragmatic hernia should be considered. Other causes of cystic parenchyma (eg, bronchopulmonary dysplasia or bacterial pneumonias with pneumatoceles) can usually be excluded by the timing of their onset.

Congenital Lobar Emphysema
Epidemiology
Congenital lobar emphysema (CLE) is the most common neonatal cause of cystic malformation of the lung. It presents within the first 6 months of life, occurs more frequently in males (1.8:1), and occasionally occurs within families. CLE usually affects the left upper lobe (50%), the right middle lobe (24%), or the right upper lobe (18%) and is frequently associated with congenital heart disease (30%), such as te-

Table 1: Causes of Partial Airway Obstruction in Congenital Lobar Emphysema

- Local bronchial cartilage deficiency resulting in redundant mucosa and bronchial wall collapse

- Hypoplasia of a segment of airway or a flap-valve formed by redundant mucosal folds

- Partial rotation of the lobe around its hilar pedicle

- External compression by blood vessels, mediastinal, or intrapulmonary masses

- Polyalveolar lobe containing an excess in alveoli and an inadequate blood supply

tralogy of Fallot, ventricular septal defect, total anomalous venous return, and patent ductus arteriosus.

Pathophysiology

Characteristically, multiple lobes of the lung contain alveoli distended 3 to 10 times normal size. This is not true of emphysema—there is no destruction of lung tissue—but rather distal overinflation of otherwise normal tissue caused by partial airway obstruction (Table 1).

Presentation

Most affected infants present with mild symptoms of airway obstruction and respiratory distress without cyanosis. Chest radiography reveals hyperinflated lobes—often herniated across the midline—and compression of the adjacent lung (Figure 1). CLE can be distinguished from other cysts, pneumothoraces, or pneumatoceles by the presence of bronchovascular markings extending to the periphery of the involved lobe and by atelectasis of adjacent tissue. Infants with pulmonary inter-

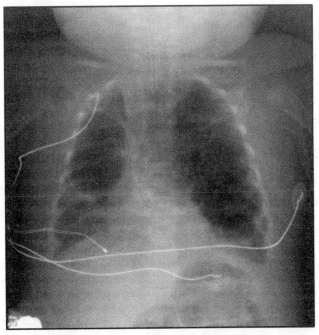

Figure 1: Radiograph of an infant with congenital lobar emphysema. Both lungs are hyperinflated with multiple, large cysts.

stitial emphysema will have a history of mechanical ventilation. Other diagnostic studies are rarely necessary.

Management

Acutely, some infants need pulmonary toilet and continuous positive airway pressure (CPAP) to maintain patency and adequate drainage. Some clinicians advocate bronchoscopy to identify and remove the source of airway obstruction. Most cases do not progress, and symptoms in mildly affected children usually resolve within a year as the severity of airway obstruction diminishes. With severe distress, lobectomy may be required.

Outcome

The long-term prognosis is excellent.

Bronchogenic Cyst
Epidemiology

The most common cause of a cyst in the lung, the bronchogenic cyst rarely presents in the neonate.

Pathophysiology

During pulmonary development, abnormal budding of the respiratory tract at any point before the alveolus produces a cyst. These cysts are lined with columnar, cuboidal, or pseudostratified epithelium and contain walls with smooth muscle and cartilage. With no communication to the airway, lung liquid secretions are trapped. Bronchogenic cysts are found predominantly in the mediastinum near the carina and are seldom large.

Presentation

This cyst produces symptoms by airway compression. Smaller cysts may be asymptomatic, incidental findings. On chest radiograph, most cysts are fluid-filled and appear as smooth, round, or oval masses. Lung distal to the compressed airway will be either atelectatic or emphysematous.

Management

Surgical excision may be necessary.

Outcome

Most cases are asymptomatic. Prognosis after resection should be good.

Neurenteric and Enteric Cyst
Epidemiology

Other intrathoracic, fluid-filled cysts (esophageal, gastrogenic, and enterogenous cysts) are extremely rare in the neonate.

Pathophysiology

They are usually located in the posterior mediastinum and are lined with gastrointestinal epithelium and layers of smooth muscle. These cysts are believed to be duplicated segments of the gastrointestinal tract that have become partially or completely detached from their parent viscera. The close association with vertebral anomalies is thought to result from common primary embryonic defects.

Presentation

Bronchial compression by the cyst may result in distal overdistention, atelectasis, or respiratory distress. Distinction between bronchogenic, neurenteric, and enteric cysts is difficult and may require computed tomography or magnetic resonance imaging.

Management

Surgical resection may be indicated.

Outcome

The long-term prognosis for normal activity and lung function is extremely good.

Cystic Adenomatoid Malformation

Epidemiology

Cystic adenomatoid malformation (CAM) is a rare cystic lesion found more often in males (1.8:1).

Pathophysiology

It is a hamartomatous lesion consisting of numerous, intercommunicating, bronchiolus-like structures of variable size with many immature cells and surrounded by a rim of lung tissue. There are three types of CAM—I, II, and III—with distinct clinical, radiographic, and histologic features.

Presentation

Polyhydramnios, prematurity, and stillbirth are common in all three types. Antenatal ultrasound diagnosis is possible.

Infants usually develop progressive respiratory distress at birth as the cysts, filling with air, cause mediastinal shift and compression of the remaining lung. A chest radiograph is usually diagnostic and demonstrates multiple, progressively enlarging cysts. Placement of a radiopaque, orogastric catheter may help to differentiate CAM from a diaphragmatic hernia. Occasionally, if the cysts grow quite large and thin-walled, CAM is difficult to distinguish from lobar emphysema or a large pneumothorax.

Management
Surgical resection is almost always required.

Outcome
When the symptoms progress rapidly, mortality is high.

Type I CAM is the most common (70% of cases) and presents as single or multiple, large (3 to 10 cm) cysts. These cysts are confined to one lobe, filled with air or fluid, and usually communicate with the bronchi. Polyhydramnios resulting from mechanical obstruction of venous return occurs in 10% of cases. Only 11% have associated anomalies. About one third of affected children present after 1 year of age, usually with cough, fever, or mild dyspnea; 90% survive.

Type II CAM is found in 18% of cases and is composed of multiple, evenly distributed, medium-sized (0.5 to 2.0 cm) cysts that resemble terminal bronchioles. It occurs in young infants, 50% of whom have other anomalies. These anomalies are often severe and include sirenomelia, renal agenesis, and extralobar pulmonary sequestration. Because of the severe, associated anomalies, only 56% survive.

Type III CAM, found in 10% of cases, is usually a large, bulky lesion with evenly distributed, small (less than 0.2 cm) cysts occupying an entire lobe or lung. This type resembles the early canalicular stage of fetal lung development and may be the result of an insult at the time of lung bud branching (26 to 28 days). Mediastinal displacement and polyhydramnios are extremely common. Associated anomalies are not described. Only 60% of infants with this condition survive.

By Karen E. Johnson, MD, and Timothy R. Cooper, MD

Other Lung Malformations

Pulmonary Sequestration
Epidemiology

Pulmonary sequestration is a rare cause of respiratory distress during the newborn period.

Pathophysiology

It represents a mass of lung tissue located within normal lung parenchyma but with an abnormal communication with the tracheobronchial tree. There are two types of pulmonary sequestration, intralobar and extralobar. Intralobar pulmonary sequestration occurs most commonly as a portion of lung within the lower lobe of a normal lung and results from chronic pulmonary infections that obliterate or obstruct the airway and normal blood supply. This sequestered lobe does not communicate with the major airways and derives its blood supply from the aorta. Recurrent infections are common.

Extralobar pulmonary sequestration (accessory lobe) consists of pulmonary tissue isolated from the lung and surrounded by its own pleura. It communicates with either the lung or gut. Occasionally familial, this sequestration has a 4:1 male predominance. More than 90% are left-sided and are located between the lower lobe and the diaphragm. About half of these children have other anomalies (Table 2), often of foregut derivation. The blood supply is from the aorta, although venous blood is occasionally provided from a branch of the pulmonary artery. Venous drainage through the azygos and hemiazygos veins results in a left-to-right shunt. Infections are less common than with intralobar sequestrations.

Table 2: Anomalies Associated With Pulmonary Sequestration

Foregut anomalies

   Tracheoesophageal fistula
   Esophageal duplication
   Neurenteric cysts
   Esophageal diverticulum
   Esophageal cysts
   Bronchogenic cysts
   Megacolon

Skeletal deformities

   Funnel chest
   Vertebral anomalies
   Polydactyly

Diaphragmatic hernias

Congenital heart disease

   Atrial septal defect
   Ventricular septal defect
   Congenital absence of pericardium
   Truncus arteriosus
   Tricuspid atresia
   Transposition of the great arteries
   Subvalvular aortic stenosis

Renal anomalies

Cerebral anomalies

   Hydrocephalus

Presentation

Both types of sequestration are usually diagnosed in childhood after a history of recurrent pneumonia. Pulmonary sequestrations appear on a chest radiograph as a unilateral, triangular or oval, posteriobasilar mass. They are usually located toward the midline. Cystic changes are common. A barium swallow may show gastrointestinal communication. Aortography demonstrates the abnormal blood supply. They must be distinguished from solid type III cystic adenomatoid malformations, bronchogenic cysts, and mediastinal tumors (neural crest tumors, teratomas, and hamartomas).

Management

Surgical resection is often required.

Pulmonary Arteriovenous Fistula

Epidemiology

A rare cause of neonatal cyanosis is abnormal vascular communications between pulmonary arteries and veins.

Pathophysiology

Single or multiple, visible or microscopic, these most commonly involve the lower lobes. Frequently, pulmonary arteriovenous fistulas are associated with skin hemangiomas or hereditary telangiectasis. Although not usually symptomatic until adulthood, arteriovenous fistulas have been reported to present in the newborn period as refractory cyanosis with a harsh murmur. Chest radiography may show a small mass lesion, but radionuclide perfusion study or digital subtraction angiography are frequently needed. The electrocardiogram may demonstrate left ventricular hypertrophy.

Management

Treatment usually involves lobectomy.

Outcome

The prognosis depends on the extent of the lesion.

Congenital Pulmonary Lymphangiectasia
Epidemiology
A rare condition, congenital pulmonary lymphangiectasia is more common in males and is occasionally familial or associated with Noonan's syndrome.

Pathophysiology
Usually there is only dilatation of the pulmonary lymphatic vessels. The condition results from either a primary developmental defect or from lymphatic obstruction. It may also be associated with lymphatic disorders at other sites or with congenital heart diseases with high pulmonary venous pressures (eg, hypoplastic left heart syndrome, total anomalous pulmonary venous return, and pulmonary venous atresia or stenosis).

Presentation
Affected infants are usually full term and present with cyanotic respiratory distress shortly after birth. On chest radiograph, the lungs are hyperexpanded with diffuse, coarse, granular densities representing dilated lymphatics. Pleural effusions are common. The diagnosis is often confused with pneumonia, pulmonary edema, or pulmonary interstitial emphysema. Confirmation of the condition is difficult and may require lung biopsy. On autopsy, the lungs are lobulated with marked dilatation of the subpleural lymphatic vessels and thick, fibrotic interlobular septa.

Management
Supportive therapy can be attempted (see *Pulmonary Edema* section, Chapter 4). There is no specific treatment for this disorder.

Outcome
In severe cases, survival of infants beyond the neonatal period is rare.

Pulmonary Agenesis

Epidemiology

Pulmonary agenesis may involve complete or partial absence of pulmonary tissue. Bilateral agenesis is extremely rare and fatal. Isolated lobar agenesis can also occur. Unilateral pulmonary agenesis is more common, may be hereditary, and is slightly more common in females.

Pathophysiology

Unilateral pulmonary agenesis usually affects the left lung and is frequently associated with other congenital anomalies (eg, VACTERL [vertebral, anal, cardiac, tracheal, esophageal, renal, and limb] association). A large variety of bronchial branching abnormalities are described, and vascular anomalies are frequent.

Presentation

Affected infants present with tracheal deviation and a nearly symmetric chest resulting from partial occupation of the contralateral chest by the remaining hypertrophied lung. The presence of breath sounds is variable. Respiratory distress and cyanosis are not often present. Chest radiograph reveals opacification and mediastinal shift into the affected hemithorax, and, in the most severe cases, increased pulmonary vascular markings on the unaffected side. The chest radiograph findings can be confused with atelectasis.

Management

Bronchoscopy, bronchography, and arteriography can be helpful in outlining the arterial and bronchial branches and in demonstrating the presence of associated cardiovascular anomalies.

Outcome

Prognosis depends on the presence of other congenital anomalies and on the capacity for sufficient pulmonary blood flow.

Table 3: Causes of Bilateral Neonatal Pulmonary Hypoplasia

Extrathoracic Compression
Oligohydramnios
Potter's syndrome
Bilateral cystic kidneys
Posterior urethral valves
Prune belly syndrome
Neurogenic bladder
Bilateral ureteropelvic junction obstruction
Atresia of urethra
Prolonged amniotic fluid leakage
Chronically elevated diaphragm—no oligohydramnios
Large abdominal masses
Massive ascites
Membranous diaphragm

Thoracic Cage Compression
Thoracic dystrophies
Asphyxiating thoracic dystrophy
Achondroplasia
Achondrogenesis
Thanatophoric dwarfism
Osteogenesis imperfecta
Ellis-van Creveld syndrome
Short-limb polydactyly syndrome
Metatropic dwarfism
Hypophosphatasia

Thoracic Cage Compression
Thoracic dystrophies (continued)
Chondrodystrophia fetalis calcificans

Camptomelic dwarfism

Spondyloepiphyseal dysplasia

Neuromuscular disease with 'functional' compression
Werdnig-Hoffman disease

Myotonic dystrophy

Amyotonia congenita

Myasthenia gravis

Decreased intrauterine breathing

Phrenic nerve agenesis or damage

Anencephaly

Intrathoracic Compression
Diaphragmatic hernia

Diaphragmatic agenesis

Chylohydrothorax

Fetal hydrops

Large intrathoracic tumor, cyst, or heart

Idiopathic

Modified from Swischuck LE: *Imaging of the Newborn, Infant and Young Child.* 3rd ed. Baltimore, MD, Williams & Wilkins, 1989.

Pulmonary Hypoplasia
Epidemiology

Pulmonary hypoplasia, which can be unilateral or bilateral, is a developmental disorder resulting in decreased numbers of alveoli, bronchioles, and arterioles. Primary hypoplasia is uncommon, and its cause is unknown. It may be seen with other anomalies.

Pathophysiology

Most infants have secondary hypoplasia of lung tissue resulting from extrathoracic compression (oligohydramnios), intrathoracic compression (congenital diaphragmatic hernia), or thoracic compression (asphyxiating thoracic dystrophy and myotonic dystrophy) (Table 3).

Infants with oligohydramnios and renal agenesis are more often severely affected, and pulmonary histology indicates developmental arrest before 16 weeks' gestation. Factors other than amniotic fluid volume are involved because the contribution of fetal urine to production is most important later in gestation. In contrast, in infants with normal renal function, the association between prolonged oligohydramnios and hypoplasia is greater when occurring before the pulmonary canalicular phase at 26 weeks' gestation.

Presentation

The neonate with extrathoracic compression usually presents with a constellation of findings similar to Potter's syndrome (Table 4). Infants with prolonged oligohydramnios from nonrenal causes virtually always have associated skeletal deformities. The chest radiograph reveals small, relatively hyperlucent lung fields. Evidence of air block is common. Abdominal ultrasound is necessary to rule out a renal or urologic cause.

Management

Ventilatory management of these infants is difficult and involves judicious use of inspiratory pressures (during initial resuscitation and later) and shortened inspiratory times to attain acceptable oxygenation (see Chapter 4). It is frequently wise to accept marginal arterial blood gas tensions and avoid additional trauma to the lungs. In addition, it is important to augment ventilator therapy with chemical alkalinization and maximize oxygen-carrying capacity and cardiac output.

Outcome

Outcome depends on the severity of the lung disease and the underlying etiology. Infants with significant pulmonary hypoplasia will almost always have positional, often transient, limb deformities. Pulmonary hypoplasia associated with renal agenesis is uniformly fatal.

By Joyce M. Koenig, MD, and Timothy R. Cooper, MD

Suggested Reading

Congenital Lobar Emphysema

Campbell PE: Congenital lobar emphysema: etiological studies. *Aust Paediatr J* 1969;5:226.

McBride JT, Wohl MEB, Strieder DJ, et al: Lung growth and airway function after lobectomy in infancy for congenital lobar emphysema. *J Clin Invest* 1980;66:962.

Shannon DC, Todres ID, Moylan FMB: Infantile lobar hyperinflation: expectant treatment. *Pediatrics* 1977;59:1012.

Bronchogenic Cyst

Boyden EA: Bronchogenic cysts and the theory of intralobar sequestration: new embryologic data. *J Thorac Surg* 1958;35:604.

de Paredes CG, Pierce WS, Johnson DG, et al. Pulmonary sequestration in infants and children. A 20-year experience and review of the literature. *J Pediatr Surg* 1970;5:136.

Ramenofsky ML, et al: Bronchogenic cyst. *J Pediatr Surg* 1979;14:219.

Neurenteric and Enteric Cyst

Superina RA, Ein SH, Humphreys RP: Cystic duplications of the esophagus and neuroenteric cysts. *J Pediatr Surg* 1984;19:527.

Cystic Adenomatoid Malformation

Bale PM: Congenital cystic malformation of the lung. *Am J Clin Pathol* 1979;71:411.

Merenstein GB: Congenital cystic adenomatoid malformation of the lung: report of a case and review of the literature. *Am J Dis Child* 1969;118:772.

Stocker JT, Dehner LP: Congenital and developmental diseases. In: Dail DH, Hammar ST, eds. *Pulmonary Pathology*. New York, Springer-Verlag, 1988, p 58.

Stocker JT, Madewell JE, Drake RM: Congenital cystic adenomatoid malformations of the lung: classification and morphologic spectrum. *Hum Pathol* 1977;8:155.

Pulmonary Sequestration

Coran AG, Drongowski R: Congenital cystic disease of the tracheo-bronchial tree in infants and children. Experience with 44 consecutive cases. *Arch Surg* 1994;129:521.

Landing BH, Dixon LG: Congenital malformations and genetic disorders of the respiratory tract. *Am Rev Respir Dis* 1979;120:151.

Nicolette LA, Kosloske AM, Bartow SA, et al: Intralobar pulmonary sequestration: a clinical and pathological spectrum. *J Pediatr Surg* 1993;28:802.

Savic B, Birtel FJ, Tholen W, et al: Lung sequestration: report of seven cases and review of 540 published cases. *Thorax* 1979;34:96.

Stocker JT: Sequestration of the lung. *Semin Diagn Pathol* 1986;3:106.

Stocker JT, Kagan-Hallet K: Extralobar pulmonary sequestration: analysis of 15 cases. *Am J Clin Pathol* 1979;72:917.

Pulmonary Arteriovenous Fistula

Dines DE, Seward JB, Bernatz PE, et al: Pulmonary arteriovenous fistulas. *Mayo Clin Proc* 1983;58:176.

Fiane AE, Stake G, Lindberg HL: Congenital pulmonary arteriovenous fistula. *Eur J Cardiothorac Surg* 1995;9:166.

Hodgson CH, Burchell HB, Good CA, et al: Hereditary hemorrhagic telangiectasia and pulmonary arteriovenous fistula. *N Engl J Med* 1959; 261:625.

Congenital Pulmonary Lymphangiectasia

Felman AH, Rhatigan RM, Pierson KK, et al: Pulmonary lymphangiectasis: observation in 17 patients and proposed classification. *Am J Roentgenol Radium Ther Nucl Med* 1972;116:548.

Laurene KM: Congenital pulmonary cystic lymphangiectasia. *J Pathol Bacteriol* 1955;70:325.

Noonan JA, et al: Congenital pulmonary lymphangiectasia. *Am J Dis Child* 1970;120:314.

Pulmonary Agenesis

Maltz DL, Nadas AS: Agenesis of the lung. Presentation of eight new cases and review of the literature. *Pediatrics* 1960;42:175.

Schecter DC: Congenital absence or deficiency of lung tissue. The congenital subtractive bronchopneumonic malformations. *Ann Thorac Surg* 1968;6:286.

Pulmonary Hypoplasia

Hislop A, Hey E, Reid L: The lungs in congenital bilateral renal agenesis and dysplasia. *Arch Dis Child* 1979;54:32.

Langston C, Thurlbeck WM: Conditions altering normal lung growth and development. In: Thibeault DW, Gregory GS, eds. *Neonatal Pulmonary Care*, 2nd ed. Norwalk, Conn, Appleton-Century-Crofts, 1986, pp 1-32.

Lauria MR, Gonik B, Romero R: Pulmonary hypoplasia: pathogenesis, diagnosis, and antenatal prediction. *Obstet Gynecol* 1995;86:466.

Perlman M, Levin M: Fetal pulmonary hypoplasia, anuria and oligohydramnios: clinical pathologic observations and review of the literature. *Am J Obstet Gynecol* 1974;118:119.

Perlman M, Williams J, Hirsch M: Neonatal pulmonary hypoplasia after prolonged leakage of amniotic fluid. *Arch Dis Child* 1976;51:349.

Swischuk LE, Richardson CJ, Nichols MM, et al: Primary pulmonary hypoplasia in the neonate. *J Pediatr* 1979;95:573.

Thibeault DW, Beaty EC, Hall RT, et al: Neonatal pulmonary hypoplasia with premature rupture of fetal membranes and oligohydramnios. *J Pediatr* 1985;107:273-277.

Chapter 7

Diseases Affecting the Diaphragm and Chest Wall

Diseases of the Diaphragm

Congenital Diaphragmatic Hernia

Epidemiology

Congenital diaphragmatic hernia (CDH) is a relatively common neonatal disorder with high morbidity and mortality. The incidence is 1:2,000 to 1:5,000 live births. Most infants with this condition are mature, two thirds are male, and in 90% the hernia is left-sided. While it is a predominantly sporadic disorder, with little or no recurrence risk, a rare familial form with a much higher recurrence risk has also been reported. CDH is associated with a high incidence of other anomalies.

Pathophysiology

Diaphragmatic hernias occur through a left posterolateral defect (foramen of Bochdalek—90%) or a right retrosternal defect (foramen of Morgagni—10%). The right side is believed to be protected by the liver during development.

The diaphragm develops anteriorly as a septum between the heart and liver. It grows posteriorly to close laterally at the foramen of Bochdalek at 8 to 10 weeks' gestation. The bowel migrates back from the yolk sac at about 10 weeks. If it arrives in the abdomen before the diaphragm has closed, a hernia results. Depending on the size of the diaphragmatic defect, the stomach as well as the small and large bowel, spleen, and liver can herniate into the chest. Pulmonary hypoplasia ensues from the resulting lung compression. Although the ipsilateral lung is most severely affected, the contralateral lung is also compressed as the mediastinum is shifted. Survival is closely related to the degree of pulmonary hypoplasia.

Pulmonary hypoplasia is manifested by a decrease in the number of bronchial generations and the number of alveoli per acinus. The number of pulmonary arterioles per square centimeter of pulmonary vascular bed is reduced. In addition, there is muscular hyperplasia of the pulmonary arterioles with abnormal extension of muscle into arterioles at the acinar level. Those vascular abnormalities place infants with CDH at high risk for severe persistent pulmonary hypertension of the newborn (see *PPHN*, Chapter 4).

Presentation

Symptoms are usually those of respiratory distress and begin in the first hours or days of life. The infant with severe symptoms may present in the delivery room with deteriorating Apgar scores, scaphoid abdomen, increased anteroposterior diameter of the chest, displaced point of maximum impulse, and breath sounds that can be decreased bilaterally or are absent on the affected side. Prenatal diagnosis of CDH is made by ultrasound demonstration of the stomach or bowel in the thorax as a fluid-filled retrocardiac mass. CDH is frequently associated with polyhydramnios. Once the diagnosis of CDH is established, it is necessary to look for other associated malformations that occur. The morbidity and mortality rates in fetuses with CDH may range from 10% to 50%. The principal advantage of prenatal detection of CDH is that it facilitates delivery at a tertiary center and immediate neonatal resuscitation. A multidisciplinary team approach should be used.

Postnatally, the diagnosis is made with a chest and abdomen radiograph (Figure 1), aided by a feeding tube placed in the stomach. This will demonstrate the hemithorax filled with a mass, usually incorporating air-filled bowel loops and the

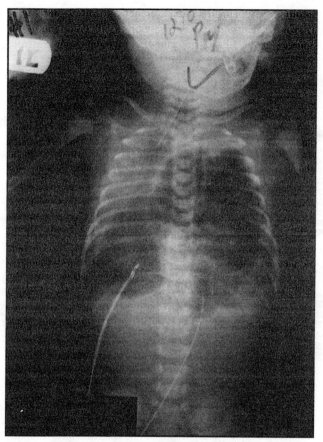

Figure 1: Radiograph of an infant with congenital diaphragmatic hernia. Multiple loops of air-filled bowel can be seen in the right chest, causing the mediastinum to shift to the left. Note there is no orogastric tube present; this should be routine. After placing the infant on intermittent gastric suction, the size of the herniated bowel was smaller and the baby easier to ventilate.

stomach within the chest. The heart is displaced to the contralateral side, and the abdomen is remarkably devoid of air.

The differential diagnosis of CDH consists of cystic adenomatoid malformation of the lung, congenital lobar emphysema, lung cyst, pneumothorax, diaphragmatic paralysis, eventration of the diaphragm, and pleural effusion.

Management

The neonate with CDH and respiratory distress from birth must be treated as a medical emergency:

- Avoid bag-and-mask ventilation by immediate intubation and ventilation. Use low peak inspiratory pressure, a rapid rate, and minimal positive end expiratory pressure (see *PPHN*, Chapter 4). Overdistention of the lungs in babies with CDH can increase pulmonary vascular resistance, causing pulmonary hypertension, and can also result in lung injury caused by barotrauma.
- Place a double-lumen orogastric tube to low, intermittent suction. This will reduce the amount of air in the hernia and further compression of the lung.
- Paralysis with pancuronium (0.05 to 0.1 mg/kg/dose IV p.r.n. movement) and sedation with morphine (0.1 mg/kg/dose IV) or fentanyl (2 to 10 µg/kg/dose IV) may be necessary to optimize ventilator support and decrease the danger of a pneumothorax. However, paralysis may lead to a loss in functional residual capacity and subsequently to a need for increased ventilatory support.
- Place an indwelling arterial catheter. Initiate noninvasive oxygen monitoring.
- If hypotension is present, provide colloid and continuous infusion of pressors, eg, dopamine (2.5 to 20 µg/kg/min IV drip).
- When respiratory acidosis is controlled, sodium bicarbonate may be used to correct metabolic acidosis.
- Evaluation for sepsis and administration of antibiotics should be considered.

- As in neonates with respiratory distress syndrome, there is both a qualitative and quantitative surfactant deficiency in CDH. Fetuses with CDH may benefit from antenatally administered maternal corticosteroids, but more studies are needed before this can be advocated. Postnatally, surfactant therapy should be considered, based on supportive evidence for surfactant deficiency in both the fetal lamb model and in human neonates with CDH. Surfactant must be used carefully, because the lungs are small relative to the infant's size. Our routine is to administer half the recommended dose of surfactant to infants with respiratory failure secondary to CDH.

The definitive treatment is surgical reduction of the hernia. There is no evidence that this is an emergency, however, and time should be spent adequately stabilizing the infant before surgery. The development of pulmonary hypertension frequently complicates the postoperative clinical course. Frequently, the patient experiences a 'honeymoon' phase, during which the infant does quite well, but then deteriorates with severe hypoxemia secondary to PPHN. The management of these infants, including special therapies such as ECMO and nitric oxide, is identical to that detailed for infants with PPHN.

Many clinicians consider ECMO for infants with CDH in whom maximal medical therapy has failed. However, ECMO is a treatment for pulmonary hypertension and not for pulmonary hypoplasia. It may succeed in improving survival by alleviating pulmonary hypertension only in those infants with an adequate amount of lung parenchyma. Patients with CDH may have pulmonary hypertension secondary to vasoconstriction or as a result of a dramatic decrease in lung parenchymal vessels. The timing of diaphragmatic repair as it relates to ECMO therapy is controversial. All proposed antenatal treatments are still experimental, and any benefits they may have over postnatal alternatives have yet to be proven.

Outcome

A multidisciplinary approach to the management of CDH—including antenatal assessment, planning, and treatment—may ensure access to state-of-the-art care to both the mother and fetus and may improve outcome.

Infants with severe respiratory distress presenting within 6 hours of birth have approximately a 50% chance of survival. In 1991, some centers suggested that ECMO might improve survival up to 60% to 65%. Various studies have suggested that a preoperative pH <7.00, Pco_2 >100, postductal Pao_2 <100, $AaDo_2$ >500, and mean airway pressure requirements >13 indicate a significant degree of pulmonary hypoplasia and very poor probability of survival.

Gastroesophageal reflux (GER) has become a significant postoperative and long-term problem after CDH repair, particularly in babies who require a large prosthetic diaphragmatic patch. This may be related to a weak diaphragmatic crus or a hiatal hernia. One study identified clinical GER in 89% of patients with CDH who underwent ECMO, and 44% of those with GER were discharged home on a regimen of nasogastric feedings. In addition, 50% of those infants treated with ECMO were at less than the 5th percentile for weight at both 1 and 2 years of age. In another study, 42% of survivors of ECMO required an antireflux operation to prevent recurrent episodes of aspiration. An aggressive multidisciplinary team approach to nutritional management in post-ECMO infants suggests improved results in adequate feeding and growth.

Paralysis of the Diaphragm

Phrenic nerve injury with diaphragmatic paralysis is a rare cause of respiratory distress. It is most commonly found after birth trauma or thoracotomy. The injuries are usually observed in large-for-gestational-age infants after shoulder dystocia or in difficult breech extractions. The nerve roots of cervical nerves 3, 4, and 5 are stretched with lateral hyperextension and traction of the neck. The diagnosis is suggested in an infant with respiratory distress, signs of birth trauma, and an elevated hemidiaphragm on the affected side. During inspiration, the affected hemidiaphragm moves up into the chest, which represents paradoxical movement. As a result, the abdominal contents often shift toward the affected side. This can be seen on physical examination as a shift in the umbilicus toward the affected side during inspiration. This has been termed positive 'belly dancer's' sign. The involved diaphragm shows either limited or paradoxical movement on fluoroscopy or ultrasound examination. Treatment ranges from no intervention to continuous positive airway pressure by nasal prongs and intermittent mandatory ventilation. Most improve over a 2-month period. If the infant continues to require mechanical ventilation, surgical plication of the diaphragm should be performed.

Disorders of the Chest Wall

Skeletal and neuromuscular abnormalities may cause respiratory distress by restriction of thoracic volume. Although bony abnormalities are rare, they may be recognized immediately and are sometimes amenable to operative correction. The severity of these disorders ranges from mild to incompatible with life.

Sternal Deformities

The most common sternal defect is pectus excavatum, an undue depression of the sternum. Rarely does this require correction unless it is progressive. Other defects of the sternum involve failure of fusion and include the following: (1) complete sternal separation, which allows protrusion of the cardiovascular structures (ie, ectopia cordis) and is commonly associated with lethal cardiac conditions; and, (2) partial sternal separation, which leads to the development of upper sternal clefts. In both situations, early surgery is required to shield the underlying structures from injury.

Thoracic Deformities

Rare skeletal defects of the thoracic cage—involving broad, short ribs, a rigid thorax, and some degree of lung hypoplasia—are part of a disease group with generalized chondrodystrophy. Asphyxiating thoracic dystrophy (Jeune's syndrome), thanatophoric dwarfism, achondrogenesis, osteogenesis imperfecta, Ellis-van Creveld syndrome (chondroectodermal dysplasia), hypophosphatasia, spondylothoracic dysplasia, and rib-gap syndrome are representatives of this group.

Respiratory distress can present at birth with severe retractions and a virtually immobile thorax. Diaphragmatic excursions are prominent, with respirations appearing entirely abdominal. Radiographically, the lungs appear airless with a diminished anteroposterior diameter. The chest has a squared-off appearance with short, clubbed ribs and a relatively large-appearing heart. A skeletal survey may help in differentiating the various syndromes. Treatment for pulmonary hypoplasia may be required (see Chapter 6).

Muscles of the chest cage may be absent and may contribute to deformities. Deficiency of pectoral muscles on one side (Poland's syndrome) may be associated with abnormal ribs and breast hypoplasia. Breathing may be paradoxical. Corrective surgery is usually done after puberty.

Muscle Weakness

Neuromuscular disorders may lead to thoracic dysfunction and respiratory failure. These primary neuromuscular disorders are usually associated with generalized muscular weakness or paralysis. These infants present with hypoventilation and a normal chest radiograph. Diseases in this group include myasthenia gravis, poliomyelitis, amyotonia congenita, muscular dystrophy, glycogen storage disease, and spinal cord injury or tumor.

By Charleta Guillory, MD, and Timothy R. Cooper, MD

Suggested Reading

Congenital Diaphragmatic Hernia

Adsick NS, Vacanti JP, Lillehei CW, et al: Fetal diaphragmatic hernia: ultrasound diagnosis and clinical outcome in 38 cases. *J Pediatr Surg* 1989; 24:654-657.

Bernbaum J, Schwartz IP, Gerdes M, et al: Survivors of extracorporeal membrane oxygenation at 1 year of age: the relationship of primary diagnosis with health and neurodevelopmental sequelae. *Pediatrics* 1995; 96:907-913.

Bloss RS, Aranda JV, Beardmore HE: Congenital diaphragmatic hernia: pathophysiology and pharmacologic support. *Surgery* 1981;89:518-524.

Breaux CW, Rouse TM, Cain WS, et al: Improvement in survival of patients with congenital diaphragmatic hernia utilizing a strategy of delayed repair after medical and/or extracorporeal membrane oxygenation stabilization. *J Pediatr Surg* 1991;26:333.

Crane JP: Familial congenital diaphragmatic hernia: prenatal diagnostic approach and analysis of twelve families. *Clin Genet* 1979;16:244.

Glick PL, Stannard VA, Leach CL, et al: Pathophysiology of congenital diaphragmatic hernia II: the fetal lamb CDH model is surfactant deficient. *J Pediatr Surg* 1992;27:382-388.

Glick PL, Leach CL, Besner GE, et al: Pathophysiology of congenital diaphragmatic hernia III: surfactant replacement for the high-risk neonate with congenital diaphragmatic hernia. *J Pediatr Surg* 1992;28:1-4.

Harrison MR, Bjordal RI, Langmark F, et al: Congenital diaphragmatic hernia: the hidden mortality. *J Pediatr Surg* 1978;13:227-230.

Langer JC, Harrison MR, Adzich NS, et al: Perinatal management of the fetus with an abdominal wall defect. *Fetal Ther* 1987;2:216-221.

Levin DL: Morphologic analysis of the pulmonary vascular bed in congenital left-sided diaphragmatic hernia. *J Pediatr Surg* 1978;92:805.

Nakayama DK, Motoyama EK, Tagge EM: Effect of preoperative stabilization on respiratory system compliance and outcome in newborn infants with congenital diaphragmatic hernia. *J Pediatr Surg* 1991;118:793.

Van Meurs KP, Newman KD, Anderson KD, et al: Effect of extracorporeal membrane oxygenation on survival of infants with congenital diaphragmatic hernia. *J Pediatr Surg* 1990;117:954.

Van Meurs KP, Robbins ST, Reed VL, et al: An early congenital diaphragmatic hernia: long-term outcome in neonates treated with extracorporeal membrane oxygenation. *J Pediatr* 1993;122:893-899.

Wilcox DT, Glick PL: Care of the fetus/newborn with congenital diaphragmatic hernia. *Fetal Maternal Med Rev* 1994;6:81-84.

Paralysis of the Diaphragm

Haller JA, Pickard LR, Tepas JJ, et al: Management of diaphragmatic paralysis in infants with special emphasis on selection of patients for operative plication. *J Pediatr Surg* 1979;14:779.

Langer JC, Filler RM, Coles J, et al: Plication of the diaphragm for infants and young children with phrenic nerve palsy. *J Pediatr Surg* 1988; 23:749.

Weisman LE, Woodall J, Merenstein G: Constant negative pressure in the treatment of diaphragmatic paralysis secondary to birth injury. In: *Birth Defects*: Original Article Series. XII, (6), pp 297-302, 1976. The National Foundation.

Chapter 8

Diseases of the Upper Airway

Disorders of the Nose, Mouth, and Pharynx

Upper airway obstruction from an intrinsic developmental defect or from secondary compression and distortion can cause severe respiratory insufficiency. The radiograph will show proximal pharyngeal distention with distal airway collapse (see Chapter 3). In contrast to lower airway disease, the lung volume is normal or subnormal.

Choanal Atresia
Epidemiology

Choanal atresia is reported to occur in 2 to 4 neonates in every 10,000 births. It has a familial tendency and a female-to-male ratio of 2:1. Two thirds of these atresias are unilateral, and 66% involve the right side. One half of affected children have associated anomalies, including Treacher Collins syndrome, tracheoesophageal fistula, palatal abnormalities, and the CHARGE association (coloboma, heart disease, choanal atresia, retarded growth and development, and genital and ear anomalies). Because 50% to 70% of children with choanal atresia have congenital heart disease, all these children should receive a cardiac evaluation.

Pathophysiology

Atresia occurs where the nasal cavity enters the nasopharynx. This obstruction may be bony (90%) or membranous. Some infants may have stenosis at the bony inlet or within

Table 1: Syndromes Associated with Pierre Robin Sequence

- Stickler syndrome
- Camptomelic syndrome
- Cerebrocostomandibular syndrome
- Persistence of left superior vena cava syndrome
- Beckwith-Wiedemann syndrome
- Myotonic dystrophy
- Radiohumeral synostosis syndrome
- Spondyloepiphyseal dysplasia congenita
- Trisomy 11q
- Fetal alcohol syndrome
- Fetal hydantoin syndrome
- Fetal trimethadione syndrome

the nasal passage, and this can result in symptoms similar to unilateral choanal atresia.

Presentation

Newborn infants are predominantly nasal breathers, so it is not surprising that nasal obstruction produces spells of cyanosis relieved by crying, as well as by mouth breathing and severe retractions. Inability to pass a 3- to 5-French feeding tube through the nares may confirm suspicions. Contrast radiographs of the nasal passage will demonstrate the level of obstruction, but computed tomography (CT) of the nasopharynx both defines the location and thickness of the obstruction and differentiates membranous from bony atresia. In the future, magnetic resonance imaging (MRI) may prove helpful.

Unilateral choanal atresia may escape detection for years. It should be suspected in infants presenting with unilateral, foul-smelling discharge on the affected side or respiratory distress associated with upper respiratory infections.

Management

Early transendonasal perforation of the atretic septum is recommended to prevent complications of intermittent hypoxia. While awaiting definitive treatment, an oral airway or endotracheal intubation may be required to maintain airway patency, and gavage feedings will be necessary. Postoperatively, nasal stints remain in place for about six weeks to maintain patency during wound healing.

Outcome

The prognosis may be poor when associated with multiple anomalies.

Pierre Robin Sequence

Epidemiology

Pierre Robin sequence (micrognathia, glossoptosis, and cleft palate) occurs once in every 2,000 live births. Inheritance may be dominant with variable expressivity. About 25% of affected children have manifestations of other syndromes (Table 1).

Pathophysiology

Mandibular hypoplasia at 9 weeks may force the tongue posteriorly, preventing closure of the palatal shelves. The cleft palate, found in 60%, is characteristically U-shaped in contrast to the typical inverted V-shape of most partial clefts. Because of the relative macroglossia, large negative pressures in the lower pharynx are created during inspiration and swallowing. This may further pull the tongue into the hypopharynx and produce pharyngeal obstruction. Recurrent episodes of hypoxia may eventually result in the development of cor pulmonale.

Presentation

The pharyngeal obstruction from this condition is usually less severe than from choanal atresia. Cyanosis is usually intermittent, especially with feedings, supine positioning, or active sleep. Chronic obstruction causes CO_2 retention, failure to thrive, and cor pulmonale. Excessive air swallowing is frequent, resulting in gastric distention, vomiting, and aspiration.

Management

Positioning the child in a prone position may clear the airway, but endotracheal intubation may be necessary to maintain an airway. A 3.5-mm endotracheal tube directed into the nasopharynx and left in place for weeks or months may be sufficient to prevent the negative pressures described above. Careful monitoring of the child (eg, multichannel tracing and home monitoring) is essential. Tracheostomy may be necessary if obstructive apnea persists.

Adequate nutrition and growth are also critical. Oral feedings may be accomplished with techniques similar to those used for infants with cleft palate. Orogastric tubes or gastrostomy may be necessary if the infant still has difficulty coordinating breathing and feeding. The palate is not usually repaired until 6 to 12 months of age.

Outcome

Generally, mandibular growth catches up with maxillary growth. In most cases, the airway obstruction resolves by 6 to 12 months, and the child develops a normal profile by 4 to 6 years of age.

Macroglossia

Airway obstruction from macroglossia may cause respiratory problems through mechanisms similar to that seen in the Pierre Robin sequence. There are many associated conditions, including trisomy 21, Beckwith-Wiedemann syndrome, congenital hypothyroidism, and large congenital tumors of the tongue (eg, hemangioma, teratoma, or lymphangioma).

Partial glossectomy or excision of the tumor or cyst may be indicated. Some hemangiomas may respond to corticosteroids.

Glossoptosis-Apnea Syndrome

Unilateral choanal atresia, choanal stenosis, or severe swelling of the nasal mucosa may generate a large negative oropharyngeal pressure. In the absence of adequate muscular control over the tongue, pharyngeal obstruction may develop.

Pharyngeal Incoordination

This condition has been observed in neonates with severe hypoxic-ischemic encephalopathy and pseudobulbar palsy, Arnold-Chiari malformation, and Möbius' syndrome. It usually produces choking and cyanosis during feedings. Aspiration pneumonia is a frequent complication. Orogastric or gastrostomy tube feedings are necessary.

Disorders of the Larynx

Laryngomalacia
Epidemiology

Laryngomalacia is relatively common, presenting at birth or within the first month of life.

Pathophysiology

This disease is characterized by easy collapse of the aryepiglottic folds, epiglottis, or larynx. The disorder occurs when poorly supported arytenoids, aryepiglottic folds, or epiglottis prolapse into the airway during inspiration.

Presentation

The condition usually presents as intermittent stridor that is influenced by position, crying, feeding, or sleeping. The stridor is inspiratory with significant chest retractions. Cyanosis, hypercarbia, abnormal cry, feeding problems, and failure to thrive are seldom present. Obstruction worsens with agitation. Radiographs of the neck may show prolapse of the aryepiglottic folds. Laryngoscopy provides the definitive diagnosis. Other conditions presenting as stridor are listed in Table 2.

Management

Conservative management is usually appropriate because spontaneous improvement is likely.

Vocal Cord Paralysis
Epidemiology

This condition is uncommon in the neonate.

Pathophysiology

Most often, unilateral paralysis occurs after injury to the recurrent laryngeal nerve. The usual causes are excessive stretching of the neck during delivery or trauma during surgical ligation of a patent ductus arteriosus. Bilateral paralysis is usually secondary to some severe central nervous system condition, including hypoxic-ischemic encephalopathy, Arnold-Chiari malformation, hydrocephalus, and brain stem dysgenesis.

Presentation

If the paralysis is unilateral, it usually involves the left side. The infant's cry is usually weak or hoarse, and stridor and retractions are not marked. Bilateral paralysis is more serious and may be associated with a characteristic high-pitched, crowing inspiratory stridor, pharyngeal incoordination, swallowing difficulties, recurrent apnea, or tracheal aspiration.

Vocal cord paralysis should be distinguished from other conditions that produce stridor (Table 2).

Management

Tracheostomy is usually needed for children with bilateral vocal cord paralysis.

Table 2: Differential Diagnosis of Stridor

Nose
Choanal atresia
Maternal reserpine
Syphilis

Mouth and Jaw
Pierre Robin
sequence
Micrognathia
Macroglossia
Hypoplastic
mandible
Thyroglossal cysts
Lingual thyroid

Larynx
Laryngomalacia
Bilateral vocal
cord paralysis
Subglottic stenosis
Laryngeal tumor
Laryngotracheo-
esophageal cleft
Laryngeal web
Reflex laryngospasm
Floppy epiglottis
Laryngeal stridor
from hypopara-
thyroidism (rare)
Calcified laryngeal
and tracheal cartilage
Laryngitis (rare)
Laryngeal infection
bacterial or viral (rare)

Trachea and Bronchi
Tracheomalacia
Tracheal stenosis
Tracheal cyst
Bronchostenosis
Bronchomalacia
Lobar emphysema

Extrinsic
Neck or mediastinal
mass
Goiter
Vascular ring
Hemangioma
Cystic hygroma
Teratoma
Tracheoesophageal
fistula

Other
Neurogenic stridor
Stridor with apneic
spells and cyanosis
Trisomy 21
Diphtheria
Neonatal tetanus

Iatrogenic
Obstruction of nares
by tubes or tape
Postintubation
laryngeal edema,
stenosis, or vocal
cord injury

Outcome

Unilateral paralysis usually improves in several weeks or months. However, bilateral paralysis has a poor prognosis that depends to a great extent on the underlying condition.

Subglottic Stenosis

Epidemiology

Acquired subglottic stenosis can be seen in 0.23% to 8% of surviving intubated babies.

Presentation

Glottic and subglottic stenosis usually result from prolonged or repeated intubation. Congenital subglottic stenosis can also occur and should be suspected if the diameter of the cricoid ring is less than 4 mm. Partial obstruction can also be caused by a laryngeal web or cyst. Supraglottic stenosis is rare. These children have inspiratory stridor with or without a hoarse cry. Soft-tissue radiography, xeroradiography, or CT are helpful, but the definitive diagnosis is made by laryngoscopy.

Prevention

Acquired subglottic stenosis is associated with endotracheal tubes that fit too snugly, with prolonged intubation, and with numerous intubations. Our policy is to always place endotracheal tubes small enough to result in an audible leak. In addition, we attempt to wean infants rapidly from mechanical ventilation to nasal continuous positive airway pressure.

Management

In mild cases, normal, spontaneous growth will often result in a sufficiently large cricoid for normal respiration. In more severe cases involving soft-tissue stenosis, an anterior cricoid split may prove beneficial. In the most severe cases, tracheostomy may be necessary while waiting for growth of the cricoid. Stenosis that results from fibrous webs, cysts, or granulation tissue can be treated with endoscopic CO_2 laser ablation.

Outcome

In most cases, symptoms from subglottic stenosis will improve spontaneously. In cases requiring tracheostomy, 2 to 5 years may be required before removal of the tracheostomy. Laryngotracheal reconstruction may then be required.

Laryngeal Tumors

Laryngeal tumors are uncommon causes of airway obstruction and stridor in neonates. The most common benign tumor of the larynx is the laryngeal papilloma, which may be induced by human papilloma viruses 6 and 11. The clinical course is unpredictable, and airway obstruction may be fatal. Diagnosis is made by visual examination with a laryngeal mirror or a flexible fiberoptic laryngoscope. Treatment is surgical and involves ablation of the tumors with a CO_2 laser. The disease tends to recur and is difficult to cure.

Additional tumors include the subglottic hemangioma (the second most frequent laryngeal mass), neurofibromas, lymphangiomas, chondromas, fibromas, and rhabdomyomas. Malignant tumors are rare but include the rhabdomyosarcoma, angiosarcoma, fibrosarcoma, chondrosarcoma, neurofibrosarcoma, and squamous cell carcinoma.

Disorders of the Trachea

Esophageal Atresia and Tracheoesophageal Fistula
Epidemiology

Esophageal atresia is a common anomaly seen in 1 in 3,000 live births. There is no sex preponderance, and 90% are associated with a tracheoesophageal fistula (TEF). About half of affected infants have multiple associated anomalies. These anomalies most often involve congenital heart disease (20%) and imperforate anus (10%) as part of the VACTERL association (which also includes vertebral, rib, renal, and limb anomalies). Many infants with Goldenhar's syndrome, CHARGE association, and trisomy 13, 18, and 21 also have esophageal atresia or TEF.

Table 3: Types of Tracheoesophageal Fistula (TEF)

Esophageal atresia with distal TEF	86%
Esophageal atresia without TEF	8%
H-type TEF without esophageal atresia	4%
Esophageal atresia with distal and proximal TEF	1%
Esophageal atresia with proximal TEF	0.05%

Pathophysiology

The esophagus and trachea first appear at the 21st day of gestation as a median ventral diverticulum of the primitive pharynx. By 34 to 36 days of gestation, lateral ridges divide the diverticulum to form the trachea and esophagus. Tracheo-esophageal anomalies occur at this stage. Five major variants of tracheoesophageal abnormalities result from abnormal septation (Table 3).

Presentation

Esophageal atresia is occasionally suspected in a pregnancy complicated by polyhydramnios. At delivery, as many as 40% of affected infants are below the 10th percentile of weight for gestational age, and 36% weigh less than 2,500 g. The diagnosis is most often made at the first feeding when the baby has difficulty from coughing, choking, and cyanotic episodes. Oral secretions are usually markedly increased. Atelectasis and pneumonia are not uncommon. The inability to pass a nasogastric tube into the stomach is diagnostic. This may be confirmed by a chest radiograph showing the tip of the tube in a wide, air-filled pouch in the upper mediastinum. Vertebral and rib anomalies may also be apparent. Contrast studies should be avoided, because the aspiration of contrast medium from a blind esophageal pouch could produce pneumonia.

On occasion, esophageal atresia without a distal esophagus to trachea fistula is suspected in an unfed infant because of a persistent airless abdomen on the radiograph. In infants with a distal fistula, the bowel may be markedly distended. The child with an H-type fistula is usually older at diagnosis and will often have a history of recurrent pneumonia; confirmation of this variant is difficult and may require contrast radiography or esophagoscopy.

Esophageal atresia is generally not difficult to diagnose. However, *H-type* fistulas may be confused with other causes of chronic pneumonitis (eg, aspiration from gastroesophageal reflux, recurrent pneumonia, cystic fibrosis, and pulmonary sequestration).

Management

Initially, continuous suctioning of the blind esophageal pouch with a double-lumen suction catheter is important. Maintain the child in a prone position, with the head of the bed elevated. In the larger newborn without respiratory distress, early primary surgical repair of the TEF without gastrostomy should be arranged. If surgery must be delayed, adequate nutritional support is essential.

In the newborn with respiratory distress, positive pressure ventilation should be avoided, if possible; effective ventilator management is difficult in infants with a distal esophagus-to-trachea fistula because of loss of airway pressure across the fistula and subsequent abdominal distention. In these infants, emergency gastrostomy and ligation of the distal fistula may be needed.

Outcome

The survival rate is excellent. Death primarily results from associated anomalies, prematurity, or low birth weight. Postoperative complications include anastomotic leaks (21%), strictures (18%), and recurrent TEF (12%). The functional outcome after primary surgical repair is good, although a few survivors have reported dysphagia.

Laryngotracheoesophageal Cleft

This is the most complete manifestation of the abnormal embryogenesis that usually leads to esophageal atresia and TEF. In this case, incomplete fusion of the tracheoesophageal septum results in a longitudinal communication between the airway and esophagus. Stridor, respiratory distress, and cyanosis are common. Surgical repair is difficult, and mortality is high.

Tracheal Agenesis

Tracheal agenesis is extremely rare, with fewer than 50 reported cases. Most cases are associated with severe genitourinary, vertebral, or cardiac anomalies. Displacement of the tracheoesophageal septum at 25 to 35 days' gestation causes failure of tracheal formation, with the bronchi arising from the esophagus. Usually, there is an associated TEF. The trachea is atretic below the vocal cords and absent to the carina. The condition should be suspected when respiratory efforts or manual ventilation fail to move air and when, on laryngoscopy, the trachea is not visualized below the larynx. Intragastric oxygen may prolong life until surgical repair can be attempted, but the prognosis is extremely poor.

Congenital Tracheal Stenosis

Congenital tracheal stenosis, which is very rare, involves a narrowed segment of the trachea, or hypoplasia of the entire trachea, with or without involvement of the bronchi. Other associated anomalies include hypoplastic lungs, vascular rings, congenital heart defects, TEF, and hemivertebra. Tracheal stenosis produces inspiratory stridor, wheezing, and, often, cyanotic episodes. The diagnosis can be suggested by a chest radiograph with air as the contrast medium. Flexible fiberoptic bronchoscopy is essential to confirm the diagnosis. Treatment varies, depending on the severity, and includes simple dilatation, segmental excision, or tracheoplasty. Mortality may be high, especially with more distal lesions.

Tracheobronchomalacia

Congenital tracheobronchomalacia is a rare disease caused by an inadequate cartilaginous framework. Secondary tracheobronchomalacia is also seen in the chronically ventilated, preterm infant. Both types can result in airway closure at some point in the respiratory cycle and may present with symptoms of stridor or respiratory distress. The diagnosis is confirmed by bronchoscopy, which shows an approximation of the anterior and posterior walls of the trachea during expiration. In the more severe cases, prolonged constant positive airway pressure may be required. The most severe cases may require prolonged tracheostomy. Fortunately, in most infants, spontaneous improvement can be expected by 6 to 12 months of life.

Vascular Rings

Table 4 shows five common anomalies that are classified as vascular rings, the first four of which result in respiratory distress.

The double arch compresses the right and left sides of the trachea and esophagus while the right arch also compresses the posterior esophagus. A right aortic arch with a persistent ligamentum or ductus results in a similar pattern of compression. The anomalous innominate artery compresses the anterior trachea only. An anomalous left pulmonary artery arising from the right pulmonary artery passes between the trachea and esophagus and is the only lesion to compress the anterior esophagus.

Infants with tracheal compression have inspiratory stridor and wheezing. Babies usually develop symptoms late in the neonatal period and often lie with their head and neck hyperextended to stretch the trachea and make it less compressible. Chest radiograph may show mild overinflation, a

Table 4: Types of Vascular Rings

Lesion	Stridor	Swallowing dysfunction	Barium swallow
Double aortic arch	Yes	Yes	Bilateral indentation of esophagus
Right aortic arch and ligamentum/ ductus	Yes	Yes	Bilateral indentation of esophagus right > left
Anomalous innominate artery	Yes	No	Normal
Anomalous left pulmonary artery	Yes	No	Anterior indentation between esophagus and trachea
Anomalous right subclavian	No	Occasional	Oblique indentation posterior esophagus

right-sided aorta, and tracheal narrowing. A barium swallow may show indentation of the esophagus. MRI or bronchoscopy may be necessary to make an accurate diagnosis. The treatment is surgical reduction of the vascular ring.

By Gerardo Cabrera-Meza, MD, and Timothy R. Cooper, MD

Suggested Reading

Choanal Atresia

Duncan NO 3d, Miller RH, Catlin FI: Choanal atresia and associated anomalies: the CHARGE association. *Int J Pediatr Otorhinolaryngol* 1988;15:129-135.

Stahl RS, Jurkiewicz MJ: Congenital posterior choanal atresia. *Pediatrics* 1985;76:429-436.

Laryngeal Anomalies

Smith RJH, Catlin FI: Congenital anomalies of the larynx. *Am J Dis Child* 1984;138:35-39.

Subglottic Stenosis

Marshak G, Grundfast KM: Subglottic stenosis. *Pediatr Clin North Am* 1981;28:941-948.

Ratner I, Whitfield J: Acquired subglottic stenosis in the very low-birth-weight infant. *Am J Dis Child* 1983;137:40-43.

Triglia JM, Guys JM, Delarue A, et al: Management of pediatric laryngotracheal stenosis. *J Pediatr Surg* 1991;26:651-654.

Tracheoesophageal Fistula

Holder TM, Cloud DT, Lewis JE, et al: Esophageal atresia and tracheoesophageal fistula. *Pediatrics* 1964;34:542-549.

Quan L, Smith DW: The VATER association. Vertebral defects, anal atresia, T-E fistula with esophageal atresia, radial and renal dysplasia: a spectrum of associated defects. *J Pediatr* 1973;82:104-107.

Spitz L, Kiely E, Brereton RJ: Esophageal atresia: five-year experience with 148 cases. *J Pediatr Surg* 1987;22:103-108.

Temtamy SA, Miller JD: Extending the scope of the VATER association: definition of the VATER syndrome. *J Pediatr* 1974;85:345-349.

Watersen BJ, Bonham Carter RE, Aberdeen E: Esophageal atresia: tracheoesophageal fistula. A study of survival in 218 infants. *Lancet* 1962;i:819-822.

Tracheal Stenosis

Dunham ME, Holinger LD, Backer CL, et al: Management of severe congenital tracheal stenosis. *Ann Otol Rhinol Laryngol* 1994;103:351-356.

Tracheobronchomalacia

Saltzberg AM: Congenital malformations of the lower respiratory tract. In: Kendig EL, Chernick V, eds. *Disorders of the Respiratory Tract in Children*. Philadelphia, WB Saunders Co, p 169, 1983.

Sotomayor JL, Godinez RI, Borden S, et al: Large airway collapse due to acquired tracheobronchomalacia in infancy. *Am J Dis Child* 1986;140:367-371.

Wiseman NE, Duncan PG, Cameron CB: Management of tracheobronchomalacia with continuous positive airway pressure. *J Pediatr Surg* 1985;20:489.

Vascular Rings

Eklof O, et al: Arterial anomalies causing compression of the trachea and/or the esophagus. *Acta Paediatr Scand* 1971;60:81.

Hendren WH, Kim SH: Pediatric thoracic surgery. In: Scarpelli EM, Auld PAM, Goldman HS, eds. *Pulmonary Disease of the Fetus and Newborn and Child*. Philadelphia, Lea & Febiger, 1978, p 166.

Wychulis AR, Kincaid OW, Weidman WH, et al: Congenital vascular ring: surgical considerations and results of operation. *Mayo Clin Proc* 1971; 46:182.

Chapter 9

Control of Breathing in Neonates

pnea of prematurity is the chief disorder of control of breathing in the neonate. It occurs in nearly 25% of preterm infants, and in 75% of those weighing less than 1,000 g. Management of this common disorder, as well as its differentiation from other pathologic states, requires understanding of the rather complex physiology of respiratory control.

Physiology

Control of breathing can be viewed as a simple feedback loop. Respiratory drive originates in a central site (the initiator), and signals are transmitted via afferent pathways to the respiratory pump mechanism (the responder). The goal is rhythmic, rather than oscillatory, breathing. Information about the response of the respiratory pump is relayed back to the initiator, and subsequent signals are adjusted accordingly. This feedback loop is facilitated by certain modifiers that promote more precise adjustment of control of breathing. These include temperature, circulation time, and carbon dioxide sensitivity. If this closed loop is opened, rhythmic breathing cannot be maintained. If modifier information is faulty or incomplete, oscillatory breathing will result as the system makes constant readjustments while searching for the correct feedback state.

Clinically, control-of-breathing disorders are characterized by various degrees of periodic breathing or frank apnea. Apnea frequency increases with decreasing gestational age, particularly below 34 weeks. Apnea may be central or obstructive, but in premature infants it is usually mixed, with about 65% central and 35% obstructive episodes.

Apnea is defined as complete cessation of breathing of 20 seconds or longer and is frequently associated with periodic breathing. Periodic breathing involves episodes of progressive diminution of rate and depth of breathing, several seconds of absent breathing, then subsequent return of respirations to baseline. Both apnea and periodic breathing may or may not be accompanied by changes in heart rate or state of oxygenation.

Central Control of Respiration

Stable control of breathing in babies is determined by three factors: central respiratory drive, maintenance of airway patency, and the respiratory pump.

The respiratory center in the brain stem is the initiator of rhythmic signals to breathe. Fetal respiratory control is characterized by periodic breathing alternating with periods of apnea. Fetal breathing is accompanied by heart rate variability as well, an important sign of fetal well-being. It is not surprising that the fetus delivered prematurely continues to exhibit periodic breathing and apnea in the postnatal state. Gestational age is the most important factor determining rhythmic respiratory control in newborns. Central respiratory drive is periodic in immature infants but improves progressively with increasing maturation. In the immature infant, certain modifiers may act to further destabilize control of breathing.

Sleep state. Control of breathing is most disorganized and periodic during REM sleep. About 65% of sleep time is REM sleep in prematures, making them vulnerable to apnea, particularly of a diurnal nature.

Temperature. A stable thermal environment promotes rhythmic breathing while thermal fluctuations promote apnea. Up to 90% of apneic episodes in prematures occur during fluctuations in the thermal environment. About 65% occur during increases in air temperature, with the rest occurring when air temperature is falling.

Chemoreceptor function. Although chemoreceptor function is present in the newborn, it is easily exhausted. Central nervous system (CNS) carbon dioxide responsiveness is blunted in immature infants. Hypoxia and hypercarbia act as central respiratory depressants, with this response persisting up to 52 weeks postconception. It is essential to maintain adequate baseline oxygenation in any infant with apnea. Drugs such as doxapram potentiate chemoreceptor function.

Circulatory time. Although poorly understood in the neonate, this is a factor in determining CNS carbon dioxide sensitivity and adaptability to changes in Pco_2.

Lung volume. The maintenance of an ideal resting lung volume (or the functional residual capacity—FRC) enhances rhythmic respiratory drive, while a low lung volume exacerbates periodic breathing and apnea. The maintenance of lung volume is one function of the respiratory pump.

Airway Patency and Airway Receptors

The upper and lower airway tree conducts the flow of respiratory gases between the environment and the alveolar-capillary interface. A complex set of neuromuscular functions and reflexes protects upper airway patency. These develop at different rates throughout gestation and may be temporarily depressed by illness or drugs. Like other components of control of breathing, maintenance of airway patency is primarily a function of gestational age but may be modified by additional factors. Disorders of upper airway function that affect control of breathing exert their effects primarily through nasal obstruction or hypopharyngeal collapse.

The nose. Newborn infants are considered obligate nasal breathers and thus depend on nasal patency for adequate ventilation. About 30% of term infants, however, demonstrate mixed oronasal breathing during both quiet and REM sleep. About 40% respond to airway occlusion with sustained oral breathing, although with reduced tidal volume. In the premature, compensatory mechanisms are poor, and nasal obstruction commonly precipitates apnea. Nasal obstruction is particularly common after nasotracheal intubation, nasal continuous positive airway pressure (CPAP), or prolonged use of nasogastric tubes.

Hypopharyngeal function. Intact hypopharyngeal function is the most important factor in the maintenance of upper airway patency in infants. The hypopharynx is a collapsible tube subjected to negative pressure during inspiration and is normally kept open during inspiration by active contraction of a system of hypopharyngeal muscles. Failure of adequate integration of this complex function leads to pharyngeal collapse, the chief cause of obstructive apnea in infants. When hypopharyngeal muscle tone is poor, the upper airway collapses at pressures only slightly below atmospheric (-0.7 cm H_2O). Integration of pharyngeal muscle function is reduced during sleep and a complete lack of resting tone may be observed during REM sleep. This increases the level of resting airway obstruction during sleep and exacerbates pharyngeal collapse during tidal breathing. Flexion of the neck further compromises airway patency. The primary effect of nasal CPAP in the management of apnea of prematurity is opposing pharyngeal collapse. Administration of xanthines may also enhance the function of the hypopharyngeal musculature.

Larynx and trachea. The larynx and trachea are more rigid than the hypopharynx and are more resistant to collapse. Laryngeal function may be impaired by immaturity, edema, or vocal cord dysfunction. Upper and lower tracheal stenosis are recognized with increasing frequency in association with intubation and ventilator management, especially suction catheter-related injuries.

The Respiratory Pump

The respiratory pump mechanism consists of the lungs, the chest cage, and the diaphragm, along with the associated intercostal muscles and accessory muscles of respiration. The respiratory pump serves two important functions in control of breathing. One is to maintain an adequate resting lung volume that facilitates rhythmic respiratory drive. An ideal lung volume also allows each breath to be taken from an efficient point on the pressure-volume curve and serves as a reservoir for continued respiratory gas exchange between tidal breaths. The pump also facilitates adequate minute ventilation and maintains normal arterial oxygen and carbon dioxide tensions, thus providing normal chemoreceptor feedback for rhythmic central respiratory drive. Function of the respiratory pump is closely related to gestational age, with immaturity of the mechanism being a major contributor to apnea of prematurity.

Bony thorax. Ribs are rigid structures that lift the chest cage and expand its volume when the intercostal muscles contract during inspiration. In the immature infant, ribs are thin and poorly mineralized. These pliable structures are unable to resist the retractive forces of the lung and chest wall and thus fail to maintain an adequate resting lung volume, adequate tidal volume, or effective distribution of ventilation.

The intercostal muscles. These muscles contract to expand the chest cage during inspiration. In addition, they maintain resting tone at end expiration to promote the continuous negative pleural pressure necessary to maintain functional residual capacity. This mechanism is disorganized during REM sleep in premature infants, resulting in loss of chest wall stability, loss of lung volume, and exacerbation of apnea. These effects of immaturity can be opposed by the use of CPAP and xanthines.

The diaphragm. The diaphragm, in conjunction with the rib cage and intercostal muscles, promotes uniform expansion of the internal thoracic volume. This promotes efficient tidal breathing and distribution of ventilation. Function of the diaphragm may be impaired by reduction in muscle mass or contractile strength, by the supine posture, or by REM sleep in small prematures. Strength of contraction and efficiency of resting tone are enhanced by xanthines.

Table 1: Conditions That Can Destabilize Control of Breathing in the Neonate

- Hypoxemia
- Septicemia
- Antepartum magnesium sulfate
- Fetal asphyxia
- Congenital anomalies of the CNS
- Intracranial hemorrhage
- Prostaglandin E infusion
- Antepartum narcotics or general anesthesia
- Metabolic disease (eg, hypoglycemia, urea cycle disorder, organic aciduria, medium-chain acyl-CoA dehydrogenase deficiency)

Differential Diagnosis of Apnea

Apnea of prematurity is the most common control-of-breathing disorder in the neonate, but other pathologic conditions must be considered when apnea occurs, especially in mature infants. If a previously stable preterm infant begins having frequent episodes of apnea, the conditions noted in Table 1 must be considered. Such infants should be promptly evaluated for stability of the thermal environment, adequacy of resting oxygenation, and the status of hemoglobin concentration and caffeine or theophylline levels. If no obvious abnormality is found, infection should be strongly suspected. Apnea in a term infant is considered pathologic and always deserves investigation.

Management of Apnea

Central respiratory drive and maintenance of upper airway patency are poorly integrated in infants less than 32 to 34 weeks' gestation. Thus, the incidence of apnea is high in such infants, and little improvement can be expected until further maturation occurs. In the meantime, these infants are extremely vulnerable to the effects of the modifying conditions discussed above. Even at a postconceptional age of 34 to 36 weeks, the introduction of feeding may be accompanied by hypoxemia, cyanosis, and bradycardia. These are not episodes of apnea, and they occur during the waking state. They do, however, involve the same immature pharyngeal mechanisms that contribute to obstructive apnea and, like apnea, they improve with maturation.

Improved understanding of control of breathing in infants has led to the introduction of effective management tools. These are particularly effective in dealing with apnea of prematurity. Decisions to treat are based on frequency of episodes and whether they produce bradycardia or hypoxemia, or require significant intervention.

General measures. All infants with apnea should be nursed in a stable thermal environment, which is best provided by a servocontrolled radiant warmer or incubator. It is critical to avoid flexion of the neck and airway closure. Adequate baseline oxygenation must be assured in the infant with apnea, both during waking and sleep. This can be done by placing the infant on a TcPo$_2$ monitor or pulse oximeter with a strip recording for several hours and noting specific events. Low-flow supplemental oxygen may be needed in some infants with apnea, but hyperoxemia must be avoided. Nasal patency must be maintained.

Xanthines. These agents enhance rhythmic respiratory drive, improve carbon dioxide response, reduce REM sleep, enhance resting pharyngeal muscle tone, and strengthen force of contraction of the diaphragm. They exert effects on almost all components of the control-of-breathing loop. There is a linear dose-response relationship for these agents, with decreasing frequency of apnea as serum level increases. More than 75% of episodes of apnea of prematurity can be abolished or significantly modified by xanthine therapy alone.

Table 2: Comparison of Methylxanthines

	Theophylline Aminophylline	Caffeine citrate
Mechanism	Increase respiratory rate and tidal volume	Increases respiratory rate and minute ventilation
Route	IV: aminophylline PO: theophylline	IV: caffeine PO: caffeine
Loading dose	5 mg/kg	20 mg/kg
Starting maintenance dose	2 mg/kg/dose q 6-8 h	5 mg/kg/dose qd
Therapeutic range	Narrow: 7-13 mg/L	Wide: 5-25 mg/L
Approximate half-life	20 hours	100 hours
Time to steady state	5 days	14 days
Side effects	Tachycardia Irritability GI intolerance	Rare

Theophylline and aminophylline. These methylxanthines increase respiratory rate and tidal volume but their effect on respiratory rate is greater. They increase heart rate as well (see Table 2 for doses and side effects). Serum levels should be monitored once steady state is achieved. Therapeutic range is 7 to 13 mg/L with increasing control of apnea as levels increase. Because of a narrow therapeutic index, side effects or signs of toxicity may be seen at or above levels of 14 to 16 mg/L.

Caffeine citrate. Caffeine increases respiratory rate and minute ventilation with little effect on tidal volume or heart rate. It has the benefits of long half-life, wide therapeutic index, and reduced cardiovascular effects. Side effects commonly seen with theophylline (tachycardia, arousal, and gastrointestinal intolerance) are rare with caffeine.

Doxapram. Doxapram is an analeptic agent with potent respiratory and CNS stimulant properties. The drug potentiates peripheral chemoreceptor activity. It is administered by continuous IV infusion at dosages of 0.5 to 2.5 mg/kg/h. At infusion rates greater than 1.5 mg/kg/h, the incidence of hypertension and central nervous system symptoms increases significantly. Because of potential toxicity, doxapram should be reserved for infants with refractory apnea of prematurity who fail other measures.

Nasal CPAP. Nasal CPAP reduces the incidence of obstructive apnea in prematures by opposing pharyngeal collapse. Central respiratory drive may also be enhanced by alterations in the Hering-Breuer deflation reflex. The technique also aids in maintaining an adequate resting lung volume. Nasal CPAP is effective in controlling about one third of apneic episodes in prematures, and does so without the potential side effects of an endotracheal tube. Nasal CPAP is most effectively delivered using short, Silastic, double nasal prongs that minimize nasal trauma and have the lowest flow resistance. CPAP should be initiated with 5 to 6 cm H_2O pressure and system flow rates of 5 L/min. Pressures can be increased progressively up to a maximum of 10 to 12 cm H_2O as needed to achieve adequate control of breathing. Changing of tubes and nasal suctioning should be minimized. Some immature infants requiring CPAP for control of apnea continue to need it until they reach a gestational age of 32 to 34 weeks, when pharyngeal muscle control usually matures.

Anemia. Anemia, particularly the progressive physiologic anemia of prematurity, may be associated with increased frequency or severity of apnea. Transfusion of packed red blood cells reduces the frequency of apnea in many prematures, although neither the incidence of apnea nor the response to transfusion is related to the hematocrit or the severity of anemia.

By James M. Adams, MD

Suggested Reading

Czervinske M, Durbin CG, Gall TJ: Resistance to gas flow across 14 CPAP devices for newborns. *Respir Care* 1986;31:18.

Martin RJ, Miller MJ, Waldemar CA: Pathogenesis of apnea in preterm infants. *J Pediatr* 1986;109:733.

Martin RJ, Nearman HS, Katona PG, et al: The effect of a low continuous positive airway pressure on the reflex control of respiration in the preterm infant. *J Pediatr* 1977;90:976.

Mathew OP: Maintenance of upper airway patency. *J Pediatr* 1985;106:863.

Miller MJ, Waldemar CA, Martin RJ: Continuous positive airway pressure selectively reduces obstructive apnea in preterm infants. *J Pediatr* 1985;106:91.

Muttitt SC, Tierney AJ, Finer NN: The dose response of theophylline in the treatment of apnea of prematurity. *J Pediatr* 1988;112:115.

Perlstein PH, Edwards NK, Sutherland JM: Apnea in premature infants and incubator-air-temperature changes. *N Engl J Med* 1970;282:461.

Wilson SL, Thach BT, Brouillette RT, et al: Influence of upper airway pressure and posture. *J Appl Physiol* 1980;48:500.

Chapter 10

Respiratory Therapy — General Considerations

Initial Stabilization

Inadequate transition from fetal to neonatal life is one of the most common causes of respiratory insufficiency in the newborn. Birth is a complicated process that requires the infant to make the transition from:

- a thermally stable environment to a relatively cold one;
- the placenta as the major organ of gas exchange to the lung;
- the parallel circulation of the fetal heart to the series circulation of the adult;
- a continuous placental source of nutrition to an intermittent enteral one.

Thermal Transition

Remember that the newborn baby is wet and naked. Its attempts to generate heat use up oxygen and glucose, both of which may be in short supply. Place the baby on a radiant warmer and dry the baby off with warmed towels. Drying can also act as a stimulus to the mildly depressed infant. When drying the extremely delicate skin of the premature infant, gently dab the skin to prevent abrasions.

Respiratory Transition

The conducting pathway for air exchange must be clear, and the mechanics for moving air in and out of the lungs must be functioning.

Table 1: Indications for Intubation (AHA/AAP Guidelines)

- Prolonged positive-pressure ventilation
- Ineffective bag-and-mask ventilation
- Requirement for chest compressions for circulatory support
- Requirement for tracheal suctioning (see meconium aspiration)
- Congenital diaphragmatic hernia

Establish the airway. Secretions of fetal lung fluid, meconium, or amniotic fluid should be removed with brief (10 to 15 seconds) suctioning of the nasopharynx and mouth. Prolonged or repetitive suctioning can occlude the airway and stimulate a vagal reflex. The stomach contents may be aspirated after effective ventilation is established. While suctioning will be sufficient for most infants, some will require endotracheal intubation to establish a stable airway (Table 1). Some institutions, including ours, also intubate at birth all infants <30 weeks' gestation (see *Management of the Airway* section, this chapter).

Establish ventilation.
(1) Assess ventilation by observing chest movement and listening for air exchange;
(2) If inadequate, ventilate with either bag and mask or bag and endotracheal tube. *Bag-and-mask ventilation is the mainstay of neonatal resuscitation and must be practiced. Obtaining an adequate seal without injuring the facial structures of the delicate premature takes practice and attention to detail;*
(3) The bag should be compressed gently with just enough pressure to see the chest rise. As the resuscitation pro-

ceeds, the pressure required to inflate the chest should decrease as air sacs are recruited. If bag-and-mask ventilation is carried out longer than 2 minutes, an orogastric tube should be placed to empty the stomach and act as a vent;

(4) Breaths should be given at the rate of 40 to 60 per minute with 90% to 100% oxygen;

(5) Reassess adequacy of ventilation: is the thorax moving symmetrically up and down with each breath? Is air entry heard symmetrically on each side of the chest? Is the baby pink and/or is there an acceptable measurement of Pao_2 or Sao_2?

If these criteria are not met, you must:

(1) recheck the seal on the mask;

(2) adjust the position of the infant's head;

(3) check for secretions in the airway;

(4) suspect some mechanical impediment to ventilation, such as pneumothorax, diaphragmatic hernia, or chylothorax; or,

(5) if the infant required intubation, check endotracheal tube placement by direct visualization.

The vast majority of infants will establish stable ventilation in the delivery room. The single most common cause of failure is an inadequate airway. If in doubt, repeat steps 1 to 5 above.

Circulatory Transition

In most infants, heart rate and blood pressure increase with adequate ventilation and oxygenation. Circulatory support usually takes the form of chest compressions, volume replacement, or medications.

Chest compressions. Chest compressions are indicated if, after 15 to 30 seconds of positive pressure ventilation with 100% oxygen, the heart rate is below 60 or between 60 and 80 and not rising. Once the heart rate is 80/min or greater, chest compressions should be discontinued. Compressions should depress the lower one third of the sternum 1/2 to 3/4 inch and

Table 2: Causes of Persistent Circulatory Insufficiency

- Volume loss from bleeding
- Myocardial dysfunction accompanying asphyxia
- Redistribution of intravascular volume secondary to sepsis

should be consistent at a rate of 90/min with a breath interposed at 30/min for a ratio of 1:3. Compressions can be performed with the balls of the thumbs, with the hands encircling the chest, or with the tips of the middle and index or ring finger. Compressions should be stopped every 30 seconds to determine if the heart rate is greater than 80. If possible, the infant should be intubated.

Volume replacement. For infants with a clear history of blood loss or sepsis and signs of poor cardiac output including pallor and weak pulses, volume replacement with 10 to 20 cc/kg of colloid (5% albumin saline, fresh frozen plasma, or blood) is clearly justified. For the asphyxiated infant without a history of volume loss, circulatory insufficiency may be the result of poor myocardial contractility (Table 2). While administration of volume may improve cardiac output in these patients, it may also raise venous pressures and worsen pulmonary edema. Rapid volume infusions may cause surges in cerebral blood flow and increase the risk of intraventricular hemorrhage (IVH) in premature infants. For this population, correction of hypovolemia should proceed cautiously. Any infant needing circulatory support should have an umbilical venous catheter inserted. Premature infants are also particularly prone to circulatory insufficiency secondary to excessively aggressive use of high pressure or long inspiratory time ventilation (see *Lung and Heart Interaction,* Chapter 2). For these infants, therapy is directed at decreasing ventilator pressures and at judicious volume replacement.

Medications. If the infant's heart rate remains below 80 despite adequate ventilation with 100% oxygen and chest compressions for at least 30 seconds, or if the infant is born without a heart rate, then medications should be given:

(1) Epinephrine: 0.1 to 0.3 mL/kg of a 1:10,000 solution is given into the endotracheal tube or umbilical venous catheter, but never through an umbilical artery catheter. The dose can be repeated every 5 minutes.

(2) Sodium bicarbonate: 2 mEq/kg of a 0.5 mEq/mL solution over 2 minutes is given to correct documented or assumed metabolic acidosis. If the metabolic acidosis persists, the dose may be repeated.

(3) Naloxone hydrochloride: 0.1 mg/kg of this narcotic antagonist is given to infants with respiratory depression and maternal narcotic administration within 4 hours of delivery. Observe the infant closely after administration because the narcotic may have a longer half-life than the antagonist.

Neither atropine nor calcium administration is indicated in the delivery room.

Nutrition Source

If the infant requires only minimal intervention to accomplish a successful transition and has a stable cardiorespiratory system, feeding either at the mother's breast or by bottle can be initiated as soon as feasible (see *Nutritional Support,* Chapter 11). If the infant has any cardiovascular instability that might be worsened by feeding or might inhibit feeding, then start an IV infusion of glucose. Begin with 4 to 6 mg/kg/min of glucose delivery and adjust according to the initial glucose level. If the glucose is less than 40 mg/dL, give a bolus of 2.0 mL/kg of 10% glucose IV over 5 minutes. Repeat the bolus and increase the maintenance glucose delivery if repeat serum glucose levels persist at less than 40 mg/dL.

Stabilization of Infants <30 Weeks' Gestation

In our center, infants <30 weeks' gestation are treated according to a minimal stimulation protocol designed to prevent surges in blood pressure that may result in intraventricular hemorrhage. This protocol is designed to insure adequate ventilation and oxygenation, prevent apnea, and minimize noxious stimuli by reducing handling and providing adequate sedation. The individual components include:

(1) Intubate and ventilate from birth through day 3 to 7.

(2) Administer prophylactic surfactant.

(3) Insert umbilical arterial and venous catheters; use catheters for all laboratory work and infusions;

(4) Sedate with phenobarbital 20 mg/kg at birth, then 5 mg/kg/d for 3 to 7 days. Supplement with morphine sulfate 0.1 mg/kg/dose or fentanyl 1 to 3 µg/kg/dose as needed. Administer morphine slowly over 20 minutes to avoid hypotension;

(5) Infuse glucose when umbilical venous line is in place;

(6) Support circulation with cautious volume replacement delivered slowly over about 1 hour or greater. For persistent hypotension, dopamine may be started at 5 µg/kg/min and increased up to a maximum of 20 µg/kg/min;

(7) Cover the infant with plastic wrap to reduce insensible water loss and heat loss;

(8) Minimize all handling:

    a. suction only as needed;

    b. no chest physiotherapy;

    c. no daily weights;

    d. no venipunctures or heel sticks;

    e. take as many vital signs from the monitor as possible;

    f. cluster all interventions that require handling of the infant;

    g. defer any part of the physical examination not necessary to the baby's immediate well-being until after the first 3 to 7 days of life when the baby is less prone to developing an IVH.

By Alicia A. Moïse, MD, and Alfred L. Gest, MD

Oxygen Use and Monitoring

Oxygen is a primary tool in acute cardiopulmonary care and represents one of the few beneficial interventions in reducing death and morbidity in neonates. Like all such modalities, however, both risks and benefits are recognized.

Physiology (see *Oxygen Transport and Alveolar Ventilation* section, Chapter 2):

The principal goal of acute cardiopulmonary care is maintenance of adequate tissue oxygenation. Adequacy of oxygenation depends on a complex interrelationship of diffusion, transport, and circulatory factors as summarized in Table 3.

Tissue hypoxia occurs when circulatory oxygen delivery can no longer support minimal utilization. At this point, oxygen consumption falls below basal metabolic rate, anaerobic metabolism supervenes, and lactic acidemia appears. If the process continues, cell death will occur.

Oxygen Administration

Oxygen is the most frequently used drug in the neonatal intensive care unit. Its use requires a physician's order, which must state how it is to be administered and monitored. In emergency situations, oxygen may be administered in amounts sufficient to abolish cyanosis. The AAP/AHA Neonatal Resuscitation Program recommends 100% O_2 be given at 5 L/min flow, using a simple flow meter and oxygen tubing that can be connected to a manual resuscitator bag, if needed. Oxygen is administered directly by holding the tubing 1/4 to 1/2 inch from the nose of the infant. As soon as this immediate goal has been achieved, monitoring can be initiated to more accurately establish the state of oxygenation and determine further needs.

Table 3: Maintenance of Adequate Tissue Oxygenation

	Type of Hypoxia			
	Hypoxic	**Anemic**	**Hypokinetic**	**Histotoxic**
Pao$_2$	low	normal	normal	normal
Hgb	normal	low	normal	normal
Cao$_2$	low	low	normal	normal
Circulation	normal	normal	low	normal
Other				metabolic block or cell toxin

The role of oxygen in the delivery room is particularly important. At birth, pulmonary vascular resistance is high, and its subsequent fall is critical to successful postnatal cardiopulmonary adaptation. The establishment of effective ventilation and normal alveolar Po$_2$ values at birth are critical determinants of postnatal transition. Oxygen is a potent pulmonary vasodilator. If apnea or bradycardia occur at delivery, mask-and-bag ventilation should be initiated immediately. Even if spontaneous breathing is adequate, oxygen should be initiated promptly if cyanosis is present and then continued until specific monitoring clarifies the underlying state of oxygenation.

Subsequent use of oxygen can be accomplished using a variety of devices, including a head hood, a nasal cannula, or positive pressure device. In all circumstances, the inspired gas mixture should be heated and humidified. The oxygen hood is often used during the acute management of infants with respiratory distress. Its primary advantages are ease of use, precision of delivery, and availability of a wide range of

Table 4: Characteristics of Oxygen Delivery Methods

Characteristics	Hood	Cannula
Duration of use	acute*	chronic**
System flow	8-10 L/min	0.25-1.0 L/min
F_{IO_2} delivery range	0.21-1.0	0.21- 0.4
Measured F_{IO_2}	accurate	not possible
Humidification	yes	yes
Heated gas flow Temp range—incubator Temp range—warmer	yes equal to incubator‡ 36°-36.5° C	no
Maintenance required	low	moderate
Easy visibility of patient	moderate	high
Enhances bonding	no	yes
Allows infant to be fed	no	yes
Adaptable for home use	no	yes

* Preferred for infants still at risk of retinopathy of prematurity.
** Use for infants requiring chronic oxygen therapy with complete retinal vascularization.
‡ Temperatures are chosen to reduce condensation in connector tubing.

oxygen concentrations. Spontaneously breathing infants with chronic oxygen needs may be managed with a low flow nasal cannula using 100% oxygen at 1/8 to 2 L/min flow. Humidification of this system is also required. It offers the advantage of promoting parental bonding and verbal and visual stimulation. However, because of the inability to control the oxygen concentration delivered, the use of the nasal cannula represents unrestricted delivery of oxygen and is not suitable for infants at risk of retinopathy of prematurity. The nasal cannula should be reserved for delivery of low concentrations of oxygen to patients requiring oxygen therapy for prolonged periods of time after retinal vascularization is complete. Typically, these are infants with established bronchopulmonary dysplasia, especially those requiring oxygen administration at home (Table 4).

Oxygen Monitoring

When oxygen is administered, clinicians must periodically monitor inspired O_2 concentration and estimate arterial oxygen tension or content. Frequency and type of monitoring depend on the nature and severity of the disease process, birth weight, and gestational age. Monitoring is made more difficult by the fact that no clear relationship has been established between any specific laboratory value and adequacy of tissue oxygenation.

Arterial Oxygen Tension (Pao$_2$)

The arterial oxygen tension measured under steady-state conditions is now the gold standard for monitoring the status of central oxygenation. The Pao$_2$ is a particularly important measurement in the management of parenchymal lung disease. Pao$_2$ and the inspired O_2 concentration necessary to achieve it is the best clinical pulmonary function test available in the newborn because it directly reflects efficiency of gas exchange in the lung. A low Pao$_2$ or high Fio$_2$ implies very poor gas transfer, while more favorable values suggest improvement in lung function. Most sources consider 50 to 80 mm Hg to be the usual range for newborn Pao$_2$. Under conditions of the controlled nursery environment, however, a Pao$_2$ less than 50 mm Hg may be both acceptable and compatible with normal tissue oxygenation. Circulatory status and hemoglobin concentration must be considered in such circumstances.

Although universally used, Pao_2 monitoring has recognized shortcomings. Validity of values are optimal when blood gas samples are obtained from indwelling catheters under quiet, resting conditions. When percutaneous puncture is necessary (ie, in older infants), agitation may occur and values obtained may not reflect steady-state conditions. It is also necessary to appreciate that arterial Po_2 values vary considerably throughout the day in sick neonates. Intermittent sampling produces only a limited view of a single point in time.

Transcutaneous oxygen monitor. Transcutaneous ($TcPo_2$) monitors are useful for judging trends in oxygenation during management of acute lung disease. These monitors measure skin surface Po_2 (not Pao_2), which under proper conditions is closely correlated with arterial Po_2. The $TcPo_2$ sensor combines a miniature blood gas electrode with a servo-controlled heater. The sensor is applied to the skin in a way that excludes any effect of environmental air on values measured. The technique depends on heating the skin at the sensor site to 43.5° to 44.0° C. This increases the tissue Po_2 as oxygen diffuses to the skin surface. With these operating temperatures and proper calibration, skin surface Po_2 at the electrode site correlates closely with central arterial Po_2.

In certain clinical circumstances, however, correlation is poor and $TcPo_2$ may underestimate Pao_2. Such conditions include circulatory insufficiency, inadequate electrode temperature, improper calibration and lack of user expertise, patient age greater than 10 weeks (skin thickness factor), and use of vasodilator agents. Maturation and thickening of skin with increasing postnatal age limit the use of this technique largely to neonates. All of these artifacts of measurement result in underestimation of arterial Po_2.

Under usual circumstances $TcPo_2$ should be in the 40 to 80 mm Hg range. There is a time lag between measured $TcPo_2$ and Pao_2 values. As a result, oxygen concentration should not be continuously raised and lowered in attempts to 'chase' fluctuating $TcPo_2$ values. The Fio_2 and management plan selected should be designed to minimize fluctuations of $TcPo_2$ values as much as possible without constant manipulations of Fio_2.

Pulse oximeter. Pulse oximetry is useful for monitoring trends in oxygenation. This technique is less complex and does not require calibration or the level of user sophistication that $TcPo_2$ monitors do. The technique measures peripheral hemoglobin-O_2 saturation (Spo_2) which in most instances is well correlated with central saturation (Sao_2). Movement artifacts may, at times, severely limit the applicability of this technique. Artifacts of saturation measurement may also occur in the presence of high-intensity light, >50% fetal Hgb, and some radiant warmers. Pulse oximetry does not measure the Pao_2 and, thus, is relatively insensitive in detecting hyperoxemia. This is particularly important to the small premature. In acute lung disease, the range of desirable hemoglobin saturation as measured by the pulse oximeter is 85% to 95%. Under such circumstances arterial oxygen content will be acceptable and hyperoxemia will rarely occur. For older infants, see *BPD,* Chapter 5.

Capillary blood sampling. Capillary blood gas determinations have been used in the clinical setting to estimate adequacy of oxygenation, but this technique tends to underestimate Pao_2. These measurements require extensive warming of extremities (43° to 44° C), free-flowing puncture, and strictly anaerobic collection. Such conditions are difficult to reproduce in the clinical setting. For this reason, capillary sampling is not recommended as a tool for oxygen monitoring.

Summary. Oxygen administration is best carried out using a combination of monitoring techniques. Such an approach minimizes the shortcomings of each and allows a clinician the most balanced view of overall status of tissue oxygenation while optimizing patient safety.

By Joseph A. Garcia-Prats, MD, and James M. Adams, MD

Table 5: Components of the Self-Inflating Bag

Component	Function
Air inlet	Draws in air during release of bag With no reservoir, maximum F_{IO_2} is 0.4
Oxygen inlet	Connect green O_2 tubing and set flow at 8-10 L/min
	Connect O_2 source to blender for specified F_{IO_2}
Patient outlet	Connects to the mask or endotracheal tube
	May add pressure manometer via special adapter
Valve assembly	Controls the pressure pop-off of the bag
	Valve usually set to pop off at 30-35 cm H_2O
Oxygen reservoir	Connected at the air inlet to deliver F_{IO_2} of 1.0
	Always connect during emergency situations

Management of the Airway

All forms of positive pressure respiratory support require unrestricted access to the infant's airway. This access can be gained using a face mask, endotracheal tube, or nasal prongs.

Bag-and-Mask Ventilation (also see *Initial Stabilization* section, this chapter):

Indications. Ventilatory support delivered by a face mask is now reserved for emergency situations, such as the delivery room management of apneic infants. The source of positive pressure support is either an anesthesia bag or a self-inflating bag (Table 5).

Technique. Mastery of bag-and-mask positive pressure ventilation equips the physician for emergency management of infants with compromised cardiopulmonary function. Its indications are for apnea and for respiratory failure. The required equipment includes a soft face mask of the appropriate size (term and preterm) and a self-inflating bag. Proper placement of the mask over the infant's face to cover the nose and mouth (and not the eyes) takes practice and close attention. The ability to troubleshoot equipment failure in an emergency and a familiarity with each component of the self-inflating bag are important.

Endotracheal Intubation

Indications. Placement of an endotracheal tube is indicated for prolonged positive pressure ventilation for infants with respiratory failure. In addition, intubation is required in the delivery room where bag-and-mask ventilation is ineffective, if tracheal suctioning is required, or if diaphragmatic hernia is suspected (see *Initial Stabilization* section, this chapter).

Technique

Equipment: Preparation for the procedure requires proper-sized endotracheal tube (Table 6), laryngoscope and blade (usually Miller 0 or 1), suction equipment, precut tape, scissors, bag and mask, and oxygen source.

Tube placement: Many supervised intubations are required to gain proficiency. *Each attempt at tube placement should never last more than 20 seconds.* Stand at the head of the infant with the laryngoscope in your left hand, and stabilize the infant's head with your right hand. Slide the laryngoscope blade over the tongue until the tip of the blade rests in the vallecula. Lift the blade slightly to move the epiglottis out of the way and insert the tube with your right hand.

Watch the tube go through the cords to the black lines of the cord guide. The tip will be 1 to 2 cm below the cords.

Table 6: Endotracheal Intubation

Infant Weight (grams) (mm)	Tube Size Inner Diameter (cm)	Distance Lip to Tip
500-999	2.5	<7
1,000 - 1,999	3.0	7 - 8
2,000 - 2,999	3.5	8 - 9
3,000 - 3,999	3.5 - 4.0	9 - 10

Continue to hold the tube firmly at the lips and remove the laryngoscope. Note where the cm marks on the tube line up with the gum of the infant. Optimal position is 6 cm plus the baby's weight in kg following the 7-8-9 rule (ie, 8 cm for a 2-kg baby) (Table 6). *A low tube that preferentially ventilates only one lung produces the risk of unilateral lung rupture and may be more dangerous than a high tube.* Position the bevel of the tube anteriorly for optimal air flow.

Auscultate over both sides of the chest and over the stomach to insure that breath sounds are heard symmetrically over the chest. Watch for symmetric expansion of the chest with inspiration, and confirm tube position with a chest radiograph. The tip of the tube should lie halfway between the clavicles and the carina.

Tape the tube with two pieces of elastic tape, which should be wound around the tube only once. Stoma adhesive can be used to protect the skin of the face from the tape. To hold the baby and tube while another person tapes, cup the baby's head in one palm, hold the tube with the thumb and forefinger of the same hand, and then gently press the tube against the roof of the mouth with the forefinger of the other hand (Figure 1).

Precautions

Tube Position: Be very cautious about tube placement. A tube that is too low will slide in and out of one mainstem bronchus with changes in head position. This will result in

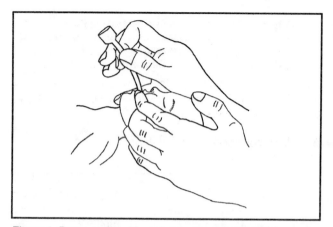

Figure 1: Proper method for tube placement. See text for explanation.

relative overinflation of one lung and may precipitate air leaks. Mainstem bronchus intubation can also lead to a maldistribution of administered surfactant, resulting in unilateral hyaline membrane disease (HMD) and unilateral lung overdistention. A tube that is too high may become easily displaced with head movements or with suctioning.

Tube Size: The size of the endotracheal tube should be appropriate for the size of the infant (Table 6) and should allow for an audible air leak. *A tube that fits too snugly significantly increases the risk of tracheal stenosis.* On the other hand, the resistance to airflow in the tube increases with the fourth or fifth power of the radius, so that small changes in tube diameter may increase resistance to gas flow substantially. These size limitations mean that it would be very difficult to deliver the high flows necessary to ventilate a 4.0-kg infant through a 2.5-mm endotracheal tube.

Type of Tube: We use orotracheal intubation in our center because of concerns about nasal deformities after long-term nasotracheal intubation and because the tip of the tube remains somewhat more stable with changes in head position.

Complications: Prolonged orotracheal intubation may cause palatal grooving and may interfere with dentition. Subglottic stenosis occurs in as many as 10% of survivors of prolonged intubation. The risk of subglottic stenosis is related to the duration of intubation, the number of reintubations, and the size of the endotracheal tube relative to the size of the infant.

Tracheobronchial Suctioning

Indications. The requirements for tracheal suctioning vary with the type of lung disease. Infants with HMD and TTN have few secretions during the acute stage of their disease. Therefore, the need for suctioning is minimal, especially since suctioning is associated with significant physiologic derangements, including hypoxia, hypercarbia, and hypertension, and may increase the risk of intraventricular hemorrhage. In this group of infants, indications for suctioning include visible secretions in the endotracheal tube, coarse breath sounds, and loss of chest wall movement while receiving mechanical ventilation. In infants with meconium aspiration or bacterial pneumonia, or in older infants with chronic lung disease, secretions can be a problem and routine suctioning is required.

Technique. Suctioning should be performed using sterile technique and using the largest catheter that fits easily down the endotracheal tube (Table 7). Suctioning through a port on the endotracheal tube adapter may prevent some of the physiologic derangements associated with suctioning. A few drops of saline instilled into the airway may help loosen tenacious secretions. Because the suction catheter can damage airway epithelium, the catheter should *not* be inserted beyond the tip of the endotracheal tube. The distance to the tip of the endotracheal tube should be recorded and posted in a convenient location at the bedside so that caregivers will know how far to insert the suction catheter. If hand-bagging accompanies suctioning, a pressure manometer must be attached to the bag to prevent delivery of excessive positive pressure.

Table 7: Considerations When Suctioning Infants

Physician's order	Indicate frequency of suctioning and special needs
Suction catheter	# 6 French for 2.5 or 3.0 tubes, # 8 French for 3.5 or 4.0 tubes
Resuscitation bag	Connect to O_2 source and to blender. Use if ventilator rate is <20/min, if infant is on CPAP, or if infant is not tolerating procedure
Wall suction	Set at continuous and at 80 mm Hg
Sterile saline	Instill 3-6 drops in tube to loosen secretions. Use either bag or ventilator for 30 seconds to distribute

Nasal Prongs

Indications. Nasal prongs are used to deliver continuous positive airway pressure. Nasal CPAP is used:

- to maintain lung volume in preterm infants with chest wall instability;
- to support the upper airway of preterm infants to prevent obstructive apnea;
- to prevent small airway closure in preterm and term infants with chronic lung disease.

Technique. A variety of nasal prongs are available for administration of nasal CPAP. Prongs must have a low resistance to gas flow and should be easy to stabilize. Flow through the system should be 4 to 5 L/min and the gas should be warmed and humidified. Excessive flow rates can cause drying or irritation to the nose or posterior pharynx. Placement and maintenance of nasal prongs can be aided by the technique in Table 8.

Table 8: Technique for Placing and Securing Nasal Prongs for CPAP

- In small premature infants, nasal prongs may remain in place better when placed upside down in the nose.

- Tape prongs in a secure manner (Elastoplast® tape works well). Do not secure prongs with occlusive bands that encircle the head.

- Position the infant's head to the side to minimize traction on the nose from ventilator tubing.

- Because prongs may be needed for a prolonged period, avoid trauma to the nose and posterior pharynx.

- Change nasal prongs only when an increased work of breathing is noticed, when sudden episodes of apnea appear, or when there are other clinical signs of nasal obstruction.

- Suction nasopharynx as needed to maintain airway patency, usually every 6 to 8 hours.

Complications. Complications are rare from use of nasal prongs. Occasional nasal deformities may result if the prongs are too large or applied too tightly. Frequent nasal suctioning may result in mucosal injury and nasal obstruction.

By Joseph A. Garcia-Prats, MD, and James M. Adams, MD

Surfactant Administration
Indications

Intratracheal administration of exogenous surfactant has been shown to reduce the severity of respiratory distress and mortality in infants. Surfactant therapy is now considered routine for treating and preventing HMD in infants.

Surfactant may be given as a prevention or prophylactic treatment or as a rescue intervention after HMD is established. Available evidence based on cost analysis and clinical outcomes such as death and pneumothorax suggests that surfactant should be given routinely as a prophylactic strategy to infants <30 weeks' gestation. When used as prophylactic treatment, surfactant should be given as soon after birth as possible. When given as a rescue treatment, a reasonable guideline is to administer surfactant when the infant reaches an arterial to alveolar oxygen (a/A) ratio of 0.22 or less. Typically, this is an infant who requires greater than 35% oxygen to maintain a Pao_2 of 50 to 80 mm Hg.

Surfactant deficiency or inactivation may be important in some forms of respiratory distress in full-term newborns. Surfactant has been used in infants with meconium aspiration and diaphragmatic hernia with encouraging results, but the studies have been uncontrolled and the number of patients involved is too small at this time to make a recommendation.

Technique Dose and Interval

Survanta®

Prophylaxis. The dose for Survanta is 4 mL/kg (100 mg phospholipids/kg) and three additional doses may be given at least 6 hours apart. Additional doses are given if the infant still requires mechanical ventilation or an oxygen requirement greater than 30%.

Rescue. The first dose is given as soon as possible after the diagnosis of HMD. Subsequent doses are administered as described for prophylaxis.

Exosurf®

Prophylaxis. The dose for Exosurf is 5 mL/kg (67.5 mg/kg colfosceril palmitate) and second and third doses may be given 12 and 24 hours later to those infants with continued oxygen or ventilatory needs.

Rescue. Two doses of 5 mL/kg are given 12 hours apart. The first dose is given as soon as possible after the diagnosis of HMD.

Techniques of Administration

The two surfactants most frequently used in the United States are given by a somewhat different technique.

The approved method of giving Survanta® involves placing a 5 French catheter into the endotracheal tube (ETT) until it protrudes slightly at the end of the endotracheal tube. Alternatively, the catheter can be placed through a neonatal suction adapter, so that mechanical ventilation is not interrupted. The surfactant is then delivered in 4 different aliquots, while the patient is placed in a different position for the delivery of each aliquot. The positions are as follows: (1) head and body inclined slightly down, head turned to the right, (2) head and body inclined slightly down, head turned to the left, (3) head and body inclined slightly up, head turned to the right, (4) head and body inclined slightly up, head turned to the left. The infant should be ventilated for 30 seconds after each aliquot.

For Exosurf®, the infant's ETT is fitted with a special ETT adapter with a sideport that is supplied with the surfactant. Therefore, the surfactant is administered without interrupting mechanical ventilation.

Exosurf® is administered in 2 half doses (2.5 mL/kg) while the infant is in midline. The instillation should be timed with inhalation and given over 1 to 2 minutes. After the first half dose is given, the baby's head and torso are turned 45° to the right for 30 seconds. Mechanical ventilation should not be interrupted. The infant is returned to the midline and the second half dose is given in an identical manner except that after the second half dose is given, the infant is turned 45° to the left.

Precautions

Prior to dosing. Ensure adequate positioning of the ETT by auscultation, visualization of chest expansion, and noting the centimeter marks on the ETT at the gum (Table 2). It is not necessary to confirm with a chest x-ray because this may unnecessarily delay surfactant administration. Any suctioning of the ETT should be performed before instillation.

During dosing.
- Monitor chest expansion. Decreased movement may represent obstruction of the airway by the surfactant. The dose may be slowed temporarily until movement returns or the peak inspiratory pressure (PIP) increases to overcome the obstruction.
- Monitor for decrease in oxygenation as determined by noninvasive oxygen monitors or visible cyanosis. Determine if chest expansion is diminished; if so, proceed as above or, if movement is good, then increase F_{IO_2}.
- Agitation may result from either of the above or the handling required for instillation. Sedation with a narcotic such as morphine may be beneficial before subsequent dosing.

After dosing.
- Pay close attention to changes in chest expansion, noninvasive oxygen monitors, and arterial blood gases for the first 30 minutes to 1 hour. Rapid changes in compliance may require frequent changes in PIP, F_{IO_2}, PEEP, and rate; otherwise, overdistention of the lung may occur, leading to possible pneumothoraces or pulmonary interstitial emphysema.
- Do not suction the patient for 2 hours after surfactant administration unless absolutely necessary.

Complications

Transient bradycardia and oxygen desaturation complicate about 10% of doses. Reflux of surfactant into the endotracheal tube, pallor, vasoconstriction, hypotension, endotracheal tube blockage, hypertension, hypocarbia, hypercarbia, and apnea occur with fewer than 1% of doses. Because of these adverse effects and the complexity and inconvenience of the approved methods of dosing, some clinicians have altered the method of surfactant delivery. It has been shown that administration of two fractional doses of Survanta® through a catheter inserted through the suction valve is as effective and safe as the current regimen that requires removal of the infant from the ventilator. Administration of Exosurf® by continuous infusion results in less loss of chest wall movement than does bolus administration. However, compelling data from experiments in animals suggest that continuous infusion may not be as effective. *Therefore, it is our policy to administer the surfactants according to the instructions on the package insert until additional efficacy data are available.*

By Alicia A. Moïse, MD, and Alfred L. Gest, MD

Positive Pressure Ventilatory Support

Positive pressure ventilatory support is used in preterm and term infants to improve oxygenation and ventilation, to support lung volume, and to prevent and treat apnea. The various types of positive pressure ventilatory support are listed in Table 9.

Continuous Positive Airway Pressure (CPAP)

CPAP is a technique for maintaining end-expiratory airway pressure greater than atmospheric pressure, ie, CPAP is positive end-expiratory pressure (PEEP) for the spontaneously breathing infant.

Physiology

In infants receiving CPAP, proximal airway pressure is usually maintained 4 to 12 cm H_2O above atmospheric pressure. This constant positive airway pressure has these physiologic effects:

Support of resting lung volume. In infants with loss of resting lung volume because of chest wall instability (see *CPIP* section, Chapter 5) or diaphragm dysfunction (eg, paralysis or eventration), CPAP increases resting lung volume and improves oxygenation and ventilation.

Table 9: Types of Positive Pressure Ventilatory Support

Continuous positive airway pressure	CPAP
Intermittent positive pressure ventilation	IPPV
Synchronized intermittent mandatory ventilation	SIMV
High-frequency ventilation	HFV
• High-frequency jet ventilation	HFJV
• High-frequency oscillatory ventilation	HFOV

Maintenance of upper airway patency. In preterm infants with poorly supported upper airways, nasal CPAP increases pressure in the posterior pharynx, prevents airway closure during inspiration, and helps prevent obstructive apnea. Similarly, in infants with chronic lung disease and damage to large central airways (trachea and mainstem bronchi), CPAP will help maintain airway patency and reduce airway resistance, particularly during expiration.

Improve distribution of ventilation. In infants with parenchymal lung disease, the lung can be divided into a well-ventilated compartment and an open but poorly ventilated compartment. Arterial oxygen tension is determined by the alveolar oxygen tension in the poorly ventilated compartment, by the size of this compartment relative to the well-ventilated compartment, and by the distribution of blood flow between the well-ventilated compartment, the poorly ventilated compartment, and the shunt (see $\dot{V}_A/\dot{Q}$ *Relationships* section, Chapter 2, and *HMD* section, Chapter 4). The only way to improve arterial oxygenation in infants with parenchymal lung disease is to improve oxygenation in the poorly ventilated compartment of the lung. Much of the ventilatory impairment in the poorly ventilated compartment is the result of increased resistance to gas flow in airways supplying these lung units. Application of continuous positive airway pressure dilates these airways, lowers resistance to gas flow, and improves ventilation. As a result, alveolar oxygen tension increases and hypoxia is relieved.

Technique

CPAP can be applied via nasal prongs or an endotracheal tube. Treatment of hypoxia in infants with severe parenchymal lung disease such as HMD often requires relatively high levels of end-expiratory pressure, 6 to 10 cm H_2O. In this group of infants, end-expiratory pressure is initially set at 5 cm H_2O with increases in increments of 1 to 2 cm to a maximum of 10 cm. While increasing end-expiratory pressure will virtually always increase Pao_2, it also overdistends the lung and may impair ventilation. If $Paco_2$ increases significantly with increased end-expiratory pressures, the infant is probably receiving too much CPAP.

The use of CPAP to prevent obstructive apnea usually requires lower levels of end-expiratory pressure, 4 to 8 cm H_2O. When CPAP is delivered by nasal prongs, there is often a flow of gas from the CPAP circuit into the nose and nasopharynx and out through the mouth. Therefore, the end-expiratory pressure in the nasopharynx and central airways will always be lower than the pressure measured at the proximal airway. The magnitude of this pressure difference will be determined to a large extent by the resistance to gas flow through the nasal prongs. With very small prongs (those used for 500- to 750-g infants) this resistance may be very high and the proximal airway pressure may have to be set high, 8 to 12 cm H_2O, to maintain even relatively modest levels of end-expiratory pressure in the airways. With CPAP delivered via an endotracheal tube, there is no flow at end expiration, and end-expiratory pressures in the central airways are similar to those measured at the proximal airway.

Precautions

The mechanical complications related to endotracheal intubation and the use of nasal prongs are described in the section on *Management of the Airway*, this chapter. Other complications related to CPAP are rare and almost all are the result of alveolar overdistention. Levels of end-expiratory pressure must be tailored to the severity of the parenchymal lung disease. If the end-expiratory pressure is too high, the more normal alveoli will be overdistended. Alveolar overdistention increases the risk of air leak and may impair right ventricular filling and blood flow through the lung (see *Lung and Heart Interaction* section, Chapter 2). An increase in $Paco_2$ with increases in end-expiratory pressure is often a warning of alveolar overdistention.

By Thomas N. Hansen, MD

Intermittent Positive Pressure Ventilation (IPPV)

The use of intermittent positive pressure ventilation has markedly improved survival for infants with respiratory failure. However, optimal use of IPPV requires the physician to have a firm understanding of how the ventilator interacts with the lung to improve oxygenation and ventilation.

Physiology

Infant ventilator. Most infant ventilators provide intermittent mandatory ventilation (IMV). In Figure 2, airway pressure (Paw) is displayed graphically over time. The infant's lungs are displayed as dashed lines increasing in volume over time. Gas flows into the ventilator circuit continuously, allowing the infant to take spontaneous breaths between ventilator breaths. PEEP is generated by a flow resistor on the exhalation limb of the circuit. A positive pressure breath is generated by closing the exhalation valve for a preset period of time, the inspiratory time (Ti), and allowing pressure to build up within the circuit. The rate at which this pressure

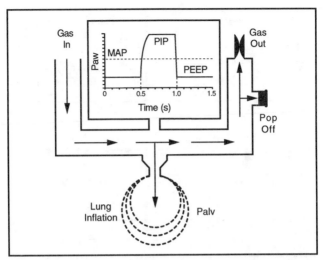

Figure 2: Time-cycled pressure-limited infant ventilator with airway pressure displayed graphically. See text for description. (Adapted from Hansen TN, Corbet AJ. In: Taeusch HW, et al, eds. *Schaffer and Avery's Diseases of the Newborn*. 5th ed. Philadelphia, WB Saunders, 1991.)

builds up is determined by the rate of gas flow into the circuit (system flow). If system flow is high, the inspiratory wave form resembles a square wave (Figure 2). The magnitude of the increase in circuit pressure is measured at the proximal airway. The maximum pressure delivered, peak inflation pressure (PIP), is limited by venting excess pressure to the atmosphere. During a positive pressure breath, airway pressure exceeds alveolar pressure (Palv), gas flows into the infant's lungs, and the lung volume increases. The respiratory rate or the number of breaths per minute is determined by both Ti and the expiratory time (Te):

respiratory rate = $60/(Ti + Te)$.

Mean airway pressure (MAP) is the average airway pressure throughout the respiratory cycle and can be increased

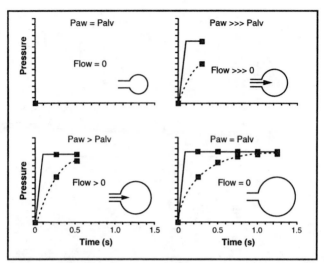

Figure 3: Determinants of gas flow into the lung. See text for description. Airway pressure Paw (solid line), alveolar pressure Palv (dashed line).

by increasing PIP, Ti, or PEEP. If the pressure wave form resembles a square wave, MAP can be calculated:

$$MAP = (PIP - PEEP) \times (Ti/[Ti + Te]) + PEEP$$

Determinants of Gas Flow Into the Lung

Alveolar pressure. Immediately before a positive pressure breath, Paw equals Palv, and there is no gas flow into the lung (Figure 3).

At the beginning of the positive pressure breath, airway pressure increases rapidly to the PIP. At this point, Paw is much greater than Palv, the driving pressure for gas flow (Paw - Palv) is large, and gas flows rapidly into the lungs. As gas flows into the lungs, the volume of gas in the lungs increases. Since Palv and lung volume are directly related (Palv = volume/compliance), as volume increases so does Palv. Therefore, over time Palv will become closer to Paw and the

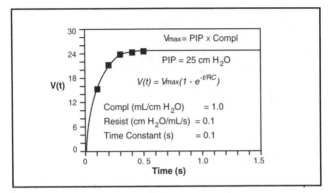

Figure 4: Lung volume above FRC as a function of time during a positive pressure breath. See text for description.

driving pressure for gas flow will decrease. Eventually, Palv will equal Paw and gas flow will cease. *The point at which Palv equals Paw marks the official end of inspiration.*

Lung volume. In Chapter 2, *Lung Mechanics*, positive pressure inflation of the lung was used as an example of a special solution to the equation of motion. While this solution does not strictly apply to the shorter inspiratory times used with conventional mechanical ventilation, Paw is still constant over much of inspiration. Therefore, the volume of gas in the lung above FRC over time is given by $V(t) = Vmax$ $(1 - e^{-t/R \times C})$ (Figure 4).

In Figure 4 the lung is inflated with a PIP of 25 cm H_2O. Obviously, at time zero, the volume of gas in the lung above FRC is zero. If inspiratory time is prolonged sufficiently (>5 time constants) then Palv = Paw, gas flow into the lung will cease, and inspiration will end. The volume of gas in the lung above FRC at this time, Vmax, is the product of PIP and the respiratory system compliance. At time points between these two extremes, the volume of gas in the lung will be determined by Vmax, hence Paw and compliance, and the respiratory time constant, hence compliance and resistance (Table 10).

Table 10: Volume Above FRC as a Function of Time for the Lung in Figure 4

Ti (sec)	Time constants	Volume % Vmax	Volume (mL)
0.1	1	63%	15.8
0.2	2	86%	21.6
0.3	3	95%	23.7
0.4	4	98%	24.5
0.5	5	99%	24.8

Increases or decreases in resistance will affect the rate of inflation but will not alter the ultimate lung volume. Changes in compliance, however, will affect the ultimate lung volume and the rate of inflation to that volume.

Determinants of Oxygenation

Cause of hypoxemia. As discussed earlier (see $\dot{V}_A/\dot{Q}$ Relationships and HMD, Chapters 2 and 4), in infants with parenchymal lung disease the arterial oxygen tension is determined by the oxygen tension in open but poorly ventilated lung units. In the case of pure $\dot{V}_A/\dot{Q}$ mismatch, continued perfusion of open but poorly ventilated lung units with very low alveolar oxygen tensions results in arterial hypoxemia. In infants with HMD, a reduction in alveolar oxygen tension in open but poorly ventilated lung units results in local vasoconstriction, redirection of blood flow through right-to-left shunt pathways, and arterial hypoxemia secondary to right-to-left shunt. In both instances, the only way to improve arterial oxygen tension is to improve alveolar oxygen tension in open but poorly ventilated lung units. *The only way for mechanical ventilation to increase the alveolar oxygen tension in open but poorly ventilated lung units is to improve their ventilation.*

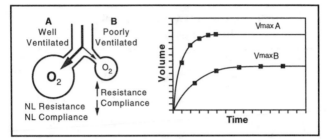

Figure 5: The illustration on the left depicts a two-compartment lung. A is a well-ventilated compartment with a normal airway resistance and compliance, while compartment B is an open but severely underventilated compartment with a reduced compliance and an increased airway resistance. In B, lung compliance is reduced so that during positive pressure inflation, the ultimate lung volume (VmaxB) is less than in the well-ventilated compartment (VmaxA). More importantly, the increase in airway resistance outweighs the decrease in compliance, so the inspiratory time constant is prolonged and compartment B inflates more slowly.

In infants with parenchymal lung disease, ventilation to open, poorly ventilated lung units is reduced because of an increased airway resistance and decreased lung compliance (Figure 5).

Effects of mechanical ventilation on oxygenation. Increasing MAP by increasing Ti, PIP, or PEEP increases arterial Po_2 in infants with parenchymal lung disease (Table 11). This implies that increasing any of the components of MAP must improve ventilation to open but severely underventilated lung units. However, as seen in Table 11, increases in PEEP are more efficient in increasing arterial oxygen tension followed by increases in PIP and finally increases in Ti. The reasons for these differences in efficiency can be understood by exploring the effects of changes in PIP, Ti, and PEEP on oxygenation (Figures 6 and 7).

Increasing MAP by increasing Ti, or to a lesser extent PIP, will result in overdistention of normal lung units (Figure 6). As discussed in the chapter on heart-lung interaction

Table 11: Efficiency of Ventilator Variables on Pao$_2$

Variable	n	Corr. Coef.	$\Delta Po_2/\Delta MAP$	P
PEEP	34	0.55	6.08	<0.001
PIP	40	0.51	5.07	<0.001
I/E	26	0.41	1.90	<0.05

MAP was increased by increasing either PEEP, PIP, or Ti, expressed as inspiratory to expiratory time ratio (I/E) in this study. For any given change in MAP, PEEP produced the greatest increase in arterial oxygen tension, PaO$_2$, followed by increases in PIP and finally by increases in Ti (Stewart, 1981).

(Chapter 2), alveolar overdistention will compress intra-alveolar vessels and divert blood flow through the right-to-left shunt. This increase in right-to-left shunt blunts the increase in oxygenation resulting from improved alveolar Po$_2$ in poorly ventilated lung units and blunts the overall increase in arterial Po$_2$. Since PEEP results in less alveolar overdistention, there is less redirection of blood flow away from well-ventilated lung units and any given increase in MAP results in a greater increase in arterial Po$_2$.

Alveolar overdistention also increases the risk of alveolar rupture and air block (see *Air Block* section, Chapter 5). Based on the discussion above, one would predict that the incidence of air block would be reduced by relying on PEEP to improve oxygenation rather than increasing Ti (or to a lesser extent, increasing PIP). In fact, several studies have now shown that methods of mechanical ventilation that use short Ti have a markedly reduced incidence of pneumothorax.

Determinants of ventilation. The Paco$_2$ is determined by the rate of CO_2 production divided by the alveolar ventilation. Alveolar ventilation is equal to respiratory rate times the difference between tidal volume and dead space volume.

Figure 6: Effects of increases in Ti and PIP on volume delivered to well-ventilated (WV) and poorly ventilated (PV) lung units. Increasing Ti from 0.2 seconds to 0.5 seconds allows more time for gas to flow into PV lung units, increasing alveolar Po_2, hence arterial Po_2. However, because of their shorter time constant, WV lung units become even more distended. Increasing PIP (dashed curves) increases the maximum volume of inflation in PV lung units, hence the volume delivered at any given Ti. The increase in delivered volume increases alveolar Po_2, hence arterial Po_2. Again,

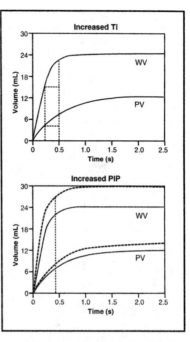

this effect is magnified in the normally compliant WV lung units, resulting in alveolar overdistention although to a lesser degree than that produced by increasing Ti. (Adapted from Hansen TN, Corbet AJ. In: Taeusch HW, et al, eds. *Schaffer and Avery's Diseases of the Newborn*. 6th ed. Philadelphia, WB Saunders, 1991.)

If dead space volume and CO_2 production are relatively constant, $Paco_2$ is inversely proportional to both the respiratory rate and the tidal volume. For the most part, tidal volume is proportional to the difference between PIP and PEEP (Figure 8).

The effects of mechanical ventilation on the $Paco_2$ are summarized in Table 12. If Ti is less than 3 time constants, increasing Ti will increase tidal volume but at the expense of overdistention of more normal lung units. It is possible to lower the $Paco_2$ by increasing the respirator rate rather than

Figure 7: Effects of increased PEEP on ventilation. Increasing MAP by increasing PEEP splints small airways open, decreases airway resistance, decreases the time constant, and allows more gas to enter poorly ventilated lung units for any given PIP or Ti. Since airways supplying well-ventilated lung units are

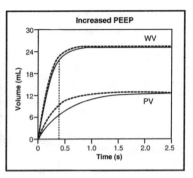

already maximally dilated, PEEP will have little effect on ventilation to this lung compartment.

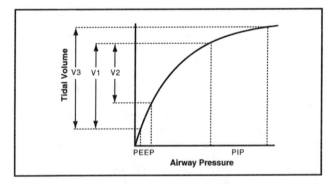

Figure 8: During positive pressure ventilation, the airway pressure cycles between PEEP and PIP. The cyclical changes in airway pressure result in cyclical changes in lung volume, the tidal volume. A plot of the pressure volume curve for the lung relates changes in pressure to changes in volume. As shown on this curve, any increase in PEEP at a constant PIP will reduce tidal volume, while any increase in PIP at a constant PEEP will increase tidal volume. However, since the pressure-volume curve tends to flatten at higher lung volumes, the ability to raise tidal volume by increasing PIP is limited. (Adapted from Hansen TN, Corbet AJ. In: Taeusch HW, et al, eds. *Schaffer and Avery's Diseases of the Newborn.* 6th ed. Philadelphia, WB Saunders, 1991.)

Table 12: Methods of Altering $Paco_2$			
	PEEP	PIP	RR
to ⇓ $Paco_2$	⇓	⇑	⇑
to ⇑ $Paco_2$	⇑	⇓	⇓

by altering ventilator pressures. However, as the respirator rate increases, the absolute time allotted for expiration decreases (see *Lung Mechanics*, Chapter 2). If expiratory time decreases to less than 3 time constants for expiration, gas trapping and alveolar overdistention may occur.

Techniques

Indications for mechanical ventilation. In our institution, >90% to 95% of infants <30 completed weeks' gestation ultimately require mechanical ventilation. Because of this and because of data suggesting that early intubation in this population reduces mortality, we routinely intubate all such infants (see *Initial Stabilization* section, this chapter). Larger infants are ventilated for apnea or for being unable to maintain a Pao_2 greater than 50 torr on a continuous distending pressure of 10 to 12 cm H_2O and 100% oxygen. We do not ventilate spontaneously breathing older infants strictly to control $Paco_2$.

Ventilator Settings

Goals of mechanical ventilation. The overall goals of mechanical ventilation are to: maintain adequate tissue oxygenation; maintain an intact circulation; and allow recovery without causing additional lung injury.

More specifically, we attempt to maintain the arterial Po_2 between 50 and 80 torr, although we will accept an arterial Po_2 between 40 and 50 torr if there is evidence of adequate oxygen delivery to the tissues. Recent evidence suggests that attempts to rigidly control the $Paco_2$ increase the risk of lung

Table 13: Initial Ventilator Settings

Rate	60
System flow	8-10 L/min
F_{IO_2}	⇑10%
Ti	0.2 SEC
PIP	25 cm H_2O
PEEP	5 cm H_2O

Typically, F_{IO_2} is set 10% greater than the patient was receiving before institution of mechanical ventilation. Ventilator gas should be warmed to 34° to 36° C and humidified to greater than 90% to prevent excessive water loss from the respiratory tract and to prevent lung injury from exposure to cold, dry air. This requires a heated nebulizer with heated ventilator circuits to prevent condensation in the ventilator tubing.

injury. We do not routinely try to lower the $Paco_2$ below 40 torr and often tolerate values of $Paco_2$ between 50 and 80 torr.

Initial ventilator settings (Table 13).

Subsequent ventilator settings (Table 14). Hypoxia should be treated initially by increasing F_{IO_2}. If this is not successful, then MAP must be increased. MAP should be increased by increasing PEEP, especially if the $Paco_2$ is not elevated (realizing that increasing PEEP will reduce the tidal volume). Increased PIP will increase both MAP and tidal volume and may be useful in those situations that require additional control of $Paco_2$. If at all possible, MAP should not be increased by increasing Ti because of the risk of alveolar overdistention and air leak. To allow sufficient time for exhalation, respirator rate is usually not increased to greater than 80 to 100 breaths/min.

Table 14:	Subsequent Ventilator Settings		
Pao_2	$Paco_2$	PEEP	PIP
low	low	⇑	
low	high		⇑
high	high	⇓	
high	low		⇓

Weaning is accomplished as shown in Table 14. For infants less than 30 weeks' gestation, when PIP is <25 cm H_2O and Fio_2 is less than 0.30, the respirator rate is slowly decreased to 15 to 20 breaths/min, and the infant is weaned directly to nasal CPAP. In this group of infants, respirator rates of less than 15 breaths/min, or endotracheal CPAP are unlikely to succeed because of the very high resistance of the 2.5-mm endotracheal tube. For the infant who cannot wean from the ventilator because of apnea or chronic lung disease, we use a respirator rate of 20 to 30 breaths/min and prolong the Ti to allow better distribution of ventilation through damaged airways (see *BPD* section, Chapter 5).

Larger infants can be weaned to endotracheal CPAP when PIP <25 cm H_2O and Fio_2 <0.40 and then to an oxy-hood when they require <5 cm H_2O of end-expiratory pressure.

Ancillary support. Endotracheal intubation and maintenance of the endotracheal tube are discussed in detail in the section on *Management of the Airway*, this chapter.

Neuromuscular blockers may shorten the course of HMD and reduce periods of non-optimal oxygenation and raised intracranial pressure associated with mechanical ventilation. In addition, there is some evidence that paralysis may reduce the incidence of intracranial hemorrhage in small preterm infants with HMD and fluctuating blood pressures (see *Lung and Heart Interaction*, Chapter 2). However, neuromuscular blockade decreases dynamic lung compliance, increases airway resistance, and removes any contribution of the infant's own respiratory effort from tidal breathing, thereby often requiring that PIP be increased. In addition, neuromuscular blockade results in significant fluid retention and makes management of fluid balance more difficult. We typically sedate ventilated infants with morphine or fentanyl and reserve neuromuscular blockade for infants requiring very high ventilator pressures (>30 cm H_2O).

Complications of Therapy

The most serious complications of mechanical ventilation are related to prolonged endotracheal intubation, air leaks, and BPD and are all discussed in those sections.

Necrotizing tracheobronchitis is a necrotic inflammatory process involving the trachea and mainstem bronchi in neonates requiring mechanical ventilation. It is thought to result from drying of the tracheal mucosa secondary to inadequate humidification in the presence of high rates of gas flow and high concentrations of oxygen. Sloughing of the tracheal epithelium with occlusion of the distal trachea causes symptoms of airway obstruction, including hyperexpansion on chest radiograph and poor chest movement. Treatment may require emergency bronchoscopy.

Atelectasis occasionally occurs after extubation from mechanical ventilation and in some instances may reflect injury to the bronchi from suction catheters. In small preterm infants, postextubation atelectasis may be prevented by weaning to nasal CPAP.

By Thomas N. Hansen, MD

Synchronized Intermittent Mandatory Ventilation (SIMV)

The frequent asynchrony of spontaneous and conventional IMV breaths in sick neonates may result in ventilator breaths out of phase with the infant's own respiratory efforts. Previous attempts to synchronize IMV breaths with spontaneous respirations (SIMV) failed because triggering devices were insensitive. In recent years, newer, more sensitive devices have been developed to detect respirations. These devices detect inspiration by measuring:

- airflow through the endotracheal tube using a hot-wire anemometer;
- airflow through the endotracheal tube using a variable orifice pneumotachometer;
- changes in chest wall impedance using a cardiorespiratory monitor;
- diaphragm movements using a balloonlike pressure capsule taped to abdomen.

SIMV systems approved by the FDA for use in newborns have a visual display that indicates spontaneous breaths and whether mechanical breaths are triggered or controlled. The delay of a triggered breath from the beginning of a spontaneous respiration is the response time in milliseconds (ms) and includes both the 'trigger' and 'system' delay. In general, response times vary between 50 and 90 ms. Most of the available systems have both SIMV and assist-control (A/C) modes. In the SIMV mode, spontaneous breaths trigger the ventilator to maintain the preset rate or to deliver controlled breaths at the preset rate during apnea. In the A/C mode, every spontaneous breath triggers a mechanical breath or delivers controlled breaths at the preset rate during apnea. In all systems, clinicians must be aware of potential problems that can increase asynchrony, including autocycling (inappropriate triggering of the ventilator due to artifact) and sensors missing spontaneous breaths.

Although some investigators have observed decreased mean airway pressure, F_{IO_2}, fluctuation of cerebral blood flow velocity, number of unit doses of sedatives and analgesic drugs, and ventilator days, claims of less chronic lung disease, intraventricular hemorrhage, or air leak syndrome have yet to be proven.

In conclusion, many systems are available that attempt to synchronize the delivery of controlled breaths with spontaneous breaths. Though these systems appear to be beneficial in some patients, their indications and benefits are not yet well defined. Clinicians who employ these systems must become familiar with their individual designs, strategies, and potential problems.

By Leonard E. Weisman, MD, and Thomas N. Hansen, MD

High-Frequency Jet Ventilation (HFJV)

The jet ventilator has been used to treat the major complication of mechanical ventilation, pulmonary interstitial emphysema, while minimizing the effect of intrathoracic pressure variations on cardiovascular function.

Physiology

For conventional ventilators, alveolar ventilation is equal to respirator rate times tidal volume minus dead space volume. HFJV achieves normal to subnormal $Paco_2$ using tidal volumes far less than dead space volume pulsed at very high respirator rates (60 to 600 cycles per second). The HFJV delivers a high-pressure 'puff' of gas through a small-bore cannula positioned in the airway at the proximal end of the endotracheal tube. These puffs of gas entrain additional gas as they jet down the center of the airway lumen. While the actual volume of gas delivered is unknown, it is clear that alveolar ventilation occurs with volumes considerably less than conventional, minimizing alveolar overdistention and air leak. Oxygenation remains proportional to mean airway pressure. Since HFJV dramatically reduces $Paco_2$ using lower mean airway pressures than conventional ventilators, it is a less effective oxygenator. In other words, use of HFJV at the low lung volumes needed to treat air block magnifies the jet's poor ability to recruit alveoli. For this reason, background conventional ventilation is often required to avoid atelectasis. The only FDA-approved indication for HFJV is for treatment of PIE, but some centers use it for infants with MAS and severe respiratory failure. Recent studies have demonstrated a poorer outcome (defined as either grade 4 IVH, cystic periventricular leukomalacia, or death) in preterm infants associated with HFJV use compared with infants managed with conventional ventilators.

Complications
Potential complications include:
- the need for reintubation with a special, larger endotracheal tube with two ports, one for delivering the jet of gas and the other for monitoring airway pressure;
- difficulty in maintaining normal FRC;
- necrotizing tracheitis (may have been minimized by newer systems of improved humidification).

By Joseph A. Garcia-Prats, MD, W. Scott Jarriel, MD, and Thomas N. Hansen, MD

High-Frequency Oscillatory Ventilation (HFOV)

HFOV was initially proposed as an alternative to conventional ventilation in an attempt to accomplish adequate oxygenation and ventilation at low tidal volumes. Although it was intended to reduce barotrauma and the development of chronic lung disease, more recently it has been used as rescue therapy where conventional ventilation has failed.

Physiology
Types of ventilators. While there are two types of high-frequency ventilators available, the strategies for their use are similar although different from conventional ventilators. One type of ventilator is the typical high-frequency oscillator that uses a piston diaphragm to actively pump gas in and out of the lung. It uses very small tidal volumes (usually less than dead space) and relies on a bias flow of gas to flush CO_2

out of the system and maintain a supply of fresh gas at the proximal end of the endotracheal tube. The operator controls frequency (3 to 18 Hz), MAP, piston displacement, and percent Ti. From these settings the operator also controls maximum and minimum airway pressure.

The other type of ventilator functions more as a flow interrupter and uses pneumatic valves to control the flow of gas in the patient circuit and generate pressure oscillations. These oscillations occur around normal IMV breaths. Although exhalation is predominantly passive, a Venturi system in the exhalation valve prevents inadvertent end expiratory pressure. The operator controls amplitude and frequency. Pressure amplitude varies around the IMV pressure that determines the mean airway pressure.

Mechanisms of gas exchange. HFOV, like conventional ventilation, increases Pao_2 by increasing ventilation to open poorly ventilated lung units. The increase in Pao_2 depends on an increase in MAP. Whether or not HFOV can produce increases in oxygen comparable to that obtained with conventional ventilators at the same MAP remains to be determined. HFOV, like HFJV, is highly effective at removing CO_2 even at tidal volumes much less than dead space volume. The rate of CO_2 removal is tidal volume dependent, and tidal volume is also frequency dependent, so that CO_2 removal is proportional to the respiratory frequency times the tidal volume squared. The mechanism by which HFOV accomplishes CO_2 removal has not been determined but there are several possible explanations:

- bulk convection of gas may occur in alveoli located near central airways;
- HFOV may facilitate molecular diffusion of gas within the terminal lung units; gas exchange may occur between lung units with uneven time constants (pendelluft);
- currents of gas flow may be set up with forward flow of fresh gas down the center of the airway and a net backward flow of alveolar/airway gas up the airway;

- enhanced dispersion of both turbulent and laminar streams of gas flow (Taylor dispersion) may occur at very high frequencies.

Indications

HMD. HFOV of experimental animals with HMD results in less lung injury than conventional ventilation. However, five randomized, controlled trials comparing HFOV to conventional ventilation have been unable to demonstrate consistent differences in mortality, incidence of air leak, or incidence of BPD. In three of these trials, the incidence of severe intraventricular hemorrhage was greater in those infants receiving HFOV.

PIE. There is some data suggesting that HFOV may be useful in treating preterm infants with respiratory failure and PIE. Like HFJV, HFOV uses very small tidal volumes and should minimize alveolar overdistention.

Term infants with respiratory failure. Some centers use HFOV to treat term infants with respiratory failure from meconium aspiration syndrome, persistent pulmonary hypertension, sepsis/pneumonia, or diaphragmatic hernia. In a single randomized trial, HFOV was more successful than conventional ventilation in reducing the need for ECMO in this patient population.

In summary, the use of HFOV for infants with HMD is still controversial. At present, HFOV should probably be reserved for treatment of preterm infants with PIE and for term infants who are approaching ECMO criteria.

Techniques

Although each ventilator has individual design and performance characteristics, the management principles are similar.

Frequency settings. The optimal frequency results in minimal pressure swings and adequate gas exchange. In preterm infants, most investigators choose a frequency range between 10 and 15 Hz.

Tidal volume. Tidal volume is determined by observing chest wall movement and measuring blood gas tensions.

Mean airway pressure. Oxygenation is determined by MAP. Typically, clinicians start with a MAP equal to or greater than that used on the conventional ventilator. MAP is increased incrementally until adequate oxygenation is achieved and the lungs appear adequately inflated on chest radiograph. HFOV is ineffective at recruiting atelectatic alveoli. Therefore, sighs must be given when the patient is initially placed on HFOV and after disconnection for suctioning. The sigh should be administered at a PIP similar to that used on the conventional ventilator.

Complications

A major concern with the use of HFOV is gas trapping. At very high frequencies, expiration may be shortened to the point that Te is less than 3 time constants, and gas trapping may occur. This may be a particular problem with ventilators that use a fixed Ti/Te. The other chief concern is the still unexplained increase in severe intraventricular hemorrhage in preterm infants receiving HFOV. Although the largest study to date appears to have primarily influenced this association, until this issue is resolved, the use of HFOV should be used cautiously in infants <31 weeks' gestation in the first 3 days after birth.

By Leonard E. Weisman, MD, and Thomas N. Hansen, MD

Nonventilatory Management of Respiratory Failure

Nitric Oxide Ventilation

Several large, randomized, controlled trials and many smaller clinical trials have suggested that inhaled nitric oxide (NO) may be a specific pulmonary vasodilator and an effective therapy for persistent pulmonary hypertension of the newborn (PPHN) by reducing the need for ECMO.

Physiology

Nitric oxide has been identified as one of the endothelial-derived mediators of organ blood flow. Disorders of NO synthesis have been implicated in many disease states, from septic shock (excess production in systemic circulation) to PPHN (inadequate production in the pulmonary circulation). The molecule is small and extremely reactive because of its free radical state. It is synthesized via the NO synthase enzyme systems by the oxidation of the guanido nitrogen of L-arginine.

The physical properties of NO make it an excellent agent for the treatment of persistent pulmonary hypertension. It exists as a gas at room temperature, and it freely diffuses through cells. Inhaled NO at very low concentrations (1 to 80 parts per million) has been shown to relax pulmonary blood vessels, thereby reducing resistance, increasing pulmonary blood flow, and improving oxygenation. The mechanism for this is the induction of guanylate cyclase, an iron-containing protein, to increase cellular levels of cyclic GMP, alter calcium permeability, and relax the cell. On the other hand, this high affinity for iron is the reason for NO's limited biologic half-life and lack of systemic effects. Once in the blood stream, NO binds tightly to hemoglobin, oxidizing the iron to form methemoglobin.

Technique

The administration of inhaled NO is still experimental and must be reserved for the extremely ill infant with impending respiratory failure. When blended into the infant breathing circuit, great care must be taken to monitor its concentration and effects. Infants should be screened with a head ultrasound and possibly with an echocardiogram before administration of inhaled NO. NO should be administered at levels ranging from 1 to 80 ppm; however, the dose response to inhaled NO appears to level out at 20 ppm. When adequate response to inhaled NO has been achieved, the dose should be actively weaned to the lowest effective dose. NO, nitrogen dioxide, and oxygen levels in the breathing circuit should be continuously monitored. It is strongly recommended that ECMO be immediately available if the infants do not respond to inhaled NO.

Precautions

The side effects of NO are related to the dose and total exposure. Methemoglobin does not usually accumulate to levels greater than 5% total hemoglobin, but can at higher doses. In cases where methemoglobin levels exceed 5%, the inhaled NO should be discontinued and consideration made for treatment with methylene blue (1 to 2 mg/kg) or ascorbic acid (200 to 500 mg/dose). Nitrogen dioxide, a compound capable of direct lung injury, can be minimized by avoiding prolonged contact of NO with oxygen before being inhaled by the patient. Its levels should be kept below 5 ppm in the breathing circuit.

Indications

Not all infants respond to inhaled NO therapy. Severe lung and circulatory disorders may limit its effectiveness. Follow-up studies will help address concerns about short- and long-term toxic effects. Until the results of these trials are known, NO therapy should be considered experimental and its use restricted to clinical trials.

By Mary E. Wearden, MD, and Michael R. Gomez, MD

Extracorporeal Membrane Oxygenation (ECMO)

Severe respiratory or cardiovascular failure in an infant that does not respond to usual aggressive medical therapy has high mortality and morbidity rates for the survivors. ECMO techniques can support an infant's ventilation and circulation, thereby allowing the condition responsible for the illness to heal.

Indications

Great care must be taken to select the appropriate candidates for ECMO therapy. In general, ECMO is most likely to be successful in infants with:

- gestational age ≥34 weeks; infants <34 weeks who are placed on ECMO and heparinized have a prohibitive risk of intracerebral hemorrhage;
- weight ≥2.0 kg; smaller infants require smaller cannulas, limiting ECMO flow;
- no preexisting bleeding disorders; systemic anticoagulation is necessary for ECMO and will be difficult to control with preexisting bleeding;
- reversible underlying disease; older infants with chronic lung diseases or conditions not likely to resolve in less than 2 weeks are less likely to benefit from ECMO;
- normal hearts; infants should have a cardiac ultrasound examination before being placed on ECMO. The presence of congenital heart disease is no longer a contraindication to ECMO. ECMO can be used to stabilize infants with anomalous venous drainage before surgery and can be used to support infants with pulmonary hypertension postoperatively.

ECMO is typically used to treat respiratory failure from: meconium aspiration syndrome; respiratory distress syndrome; pneumonia and sepsis; PPHN; and selected forms of congenital heart disease, both preoperatively and postoperatively. The benefits of ECMO to infants with congenital diaphragmatic hernia remain controversial.

ECMO criteria are designed to select those infants with a high risk of death or severe adverse outcome. Although there is some variation among the centers, criteria usually include some measure of inadequate oxygenation despite maximal support. Since ventilatory expertise and outcomes vary among institutions, each program may have to develop its own ECMO criteria. In general, these include criteria that identify infants with an 80% mortality. In our program, to be eligible for ECMO the infant must have *one of the following:*

- An alveolar to arterial oxygen difference >600 torr for 6 to 12 hours;
- Pao_2 <40 torr for more than 4 hours;
- oxygenation index (OI) >40 for more than 4 hours where the OI = (mean airway pressure) x $(Fio_2)/Pao_2$.

In addition, the infant must have some other measure of inadequate tissue oxygenation, such as an arterial pH <7.25 or arterial lactate >3.0 mmol/L on serial measures.

Technique

ECMO is not a cure for cardiorespiratory failure. It simply supports ventilation or circulation until the organs recover. There are two general techniques for ECMO: veno-arterial and veno-venous. Both techniques use the same basic ECMO system, consisting of a roller pump, membrane oxygenator, and heat exchanger connected in series and primed with heparinized blood.

For veno-arterial ECMO, a catheter is inserted in the right internal jugular vein with its tip in the right atrium, and another catheter is inserted in the right common carotid artery with its tip in the arch of the aorta. The infant is anticoagulated with a bolus of heparin and is connected to the circuit. Poorly oxygenated blood is drained from the right atrium, pumped through the ECMO system, where oxygen is added and carbon dioxide is removed, and then returned to the aorta via the right internal carotid artery, thus bypassing the entire pulmonary circulation. After connecting the infant to the circuit, the flow is slowly increased to about 150 mL/kg/min, after which the mechanical ventilator can be reduced to decrease the exposure to oxygen toxicity, barotrauma, and volutrauma. Typical settings may be 30% oxygen and low respiratory rates and peak inflation pressures so that the lung can begin to recover. The Pao_2 is maintained between 50 to 70 mmHg by adjusting the ECMO flow. The infant receives a continuous infusion of heparin to maintain the clotting time 2 to 3 times normal. Platelets are transfused to maintain the platelet count above 100,000/mm^3. After 4 to 5 days of ECMO, when there is evidence that the underlying condition is improving, the infant is weaned by gradually reducing the circuit flow while increasing the ventilator settings as needed. After a brief trial off, the infant can be decannulated. In addition to supporting oxygenation and providing for CO_2 removal, veno-arterial ECMO offers considerable circulatory support.

Veno-venous ECMO is performed by draining blood from the right atrium as well, but the oxygenated blood is then returned to the venous system either by a second cannula site or a double lumen cannula in the right atrium. This technique is not true bypass. Although it can support oxygenation and accomplishes CO_2 removal, it typically does not support circulation. Also, because of some venous recirculation, it is less efficient at oxygen delivery than veno-arterial ECMO. The advantage of veno-venous ECMO is that the carotid artery is spared.

Outcome

From 1981 through 1995, more than 13,974 infants received ECMO therapy, with a 73% overall survival in a group with a high predicted mortality. The best survival rate, approaching 90%, is with the medical conditions (meconium aspiration, pulmonary hypertension); the poorest survival rate (58%) is with the surgical condition of diaphragmatic hernia. A recent randomized, controlled trial conducted in the United Kingdom demonstrated a reduced risk of death or severe disability when ECMO was available to infants with severe lung diseases.

Complications

The most serious complications of ECMO are related to the central nervous system, with intracranial bleeding or cerebral infarcts occurring in 17% of infants. Other less frequent complications include sepsis, hemorrhage either at surgical sites or gastrointestinal, and complications related to the ECMO circuit, especially clots. Because infants who require ECMO have severe underlying cardiopulmonary disturbances, the effects on neurologic outcome are difficult to determine. Follow-up has not identified any unique complications among ECMO survivors, but only follow-up into adulthood will determine the ultimate effects of neck vessel ligation.

By Alicia A. Moïse, MD, and Michael R. Gomez, MD

Suggested Reading

Initial Stabilization

Bloom RS, Cropley C, and the AHA/AAP Neonatal Resuscitation Steering Committee, eds. *Textbook of Neonatal Resuscitation.* American Heart Association and American Academy of Pediatrics, 1995.

Disorders of the neonate. Part II: In: Winters RW, ed. *The Body Fluids in Pediatrics.* Boston, Little, Brown Co, 1973, pp 185-348.

Goddard-Finegold J: Experimental models of intraventricular hemorrhage. In: Pape KE, Wigglesworth JS, eds. *Perinatal Brain Lesions.* Boston, Blackwell Scientific Publications, 1989, pp 115-133.

Oxygen Use and Monitoring

Adams JM, Murfin K, Mort J, et al: Detection of hyperoxemia in neonates by a new pulse oximeter. *Neonatal Intensive Care* 1994;42-45.

Brunstler I, Enders A, Versmold HT: Skin surface Pco_2 monitoring in newborn infants in shock: effect of hypotension and electrode temperature. *J Pediatr* 1982;100:454.

Bucher HU, Fanconi S, Baeckert P, et al: Hyperoxemia in newborn infants: detection by pulse oximetry. *Pediatrics* 1989;84:226-230.

Clark JS, Votteri B, Ariagno RL, et al: Noninvasive assessment of blood gases. *Am Rev Respir Dis* 1992;145:220-232.

Cochran WD: Umbilical artery catheterization. In: Report of the 69th Ross Conference on Pediatric Research, *Iatrogenic Problems in Neonatal Intensive Care.* Columbus, Ross Laboratories, 1976.

Editorial: Blood gas monitors: justifiable enthusiasm with a note of caution. *Am J Respir Crit Care Med* 1994;149:850-851.

Hansen TN, Tooley WH: Skin surface carbon dioxide tension in sick infants. *Pediatrics* 1979;64:942.

Huch R, Huch A, Albani M, et al: Transcutaneous Po_2 monitoring in routine management of infants and children with cardiorespiratory problems. *Pediatrics* 1976;57:681.

Jackson JC, Truog WE, Watchko JF, et al: Efficacy of thromboresistant umbilical artery catheters in reducing aortic thrombosis and related complications. *J Pediatr* 1987;110:102.

Jennis MS, Peabody JL: Pulse oximetry: an alternative method for the assessment of oxygenation in newborn infants. *Pediatrics* 1987;79:524.

Landers S, Hansen TN: Skin surface oxygen monitoring. *Perinatol Neonatol* 1984;8:39.

Moïse A, Landers S, Fraley K: Colonization and infection of umbilical catheters in newborn infants. *Pediatr Res* 1986;20:400A. Abstract.

Neal WA, Reynolds JW, Jarvis CW, et al: Umbilical artery catheterization: demonstration of arterial thrombosis by aortography. *Pediatrics* 1972;50:6.

Poets CF, Southall DP: Noninvasive monitoring of oxygenation in infants and children: practical considerations and areas of concern. *Pediatrics* 1994;93:737-744.

Poets CF, Wilken M, Seidenberg J, et al: Reliability of a pulse oximeter in the detection of hyperoxemia. *J Pediatr* 1993;122:87-90.

Pologe JA: Pulse oximetry: technical aspects of machine design. *Int Anesthesiol Clin* 1987;25:137.

Ramanathan R, Durand M, Larrazabal C: Pulse oximetry in very low birth weight infants with acute and chronic lung disease. *Pediatrics* 1987;79:612.

Rodriguez LR, Kotin N, Lowenthal D, et al: A study of pediatric house staff's knowledge of pulse oximetry. *Pediatrics* 1994;93:810-813.

Symanski MR, Fox HA: Umbilical vessel catheterization: indications, management, and evaluation of the technique. *J Pediatr* 1972;80:820.

Wukitsch MW: Pulse oximetry: historical review and Ohmeda functional analysis. *Int J Clin Monit Comput* 1987;4:161.

Management of the Airway

Bizzle TL, Kotas TV: Positive pressure hand ventilation: potential errors in estimating inflation pressures. *Pediatrics* 1983;72:122.

Cotton RT, Seid AB:. Management of the extubation problem in the premature child: anterior cricoid split as an alternative to tracheotomy. *Ann Otol Rhinol Laryngol* 1980;89:508.

Donn SM, Blane CE: Endotracheal tube movement in the preterm neonate: oral versus nasal intubation. *Ann Otol Rhinol Laryngol* 1985;84:18.

Duke PM, Coulson JD, Santos JI, et al: Cleft palate associated with prolonged orotracheal intubation in infancy. *J Pediatr* 1976;89:990.

Fan LL, Flynn JW, Pathak DR: Risk factors predicting laryngeal injury in intubated neonates. *Crit Care Med* 1983;11:431.

Fanconi S, Duc G: Intratracheal suctioning in sick preterm infants: prevention of intracranial hypertension and cerebral hypoperfusion by muscle paralysis. *Pediatrics* 1987;79:538-543.

Greisen G, Frederiksen PS, Hertel J, et al: Catecholamine response to chest physiotherapy and endotracheal suctioning in preterm infants. *Acta Paediatr Scand* 1985;74:525.

Jung AL, Thomas GK: Stricture of the nasal vestibule: a complication of nasotracheal intubation in newborn infants. *J Pediatr* 1974;85:412.

McMillan DD, Rademaker AW, Buchan KA, et al: Benefits of orotracheal and nasotracheal intubation in neonates requiring ventilatory assistance. *Pediatrics* 1986;77:39.

Miller KE, Edwards DK, Hilton S, et al: Acquired lobar emphysema in premature infants with bronchopulmonary dysplasia: an iatrogenic disease? *Pediatr Radiol* 1981;138:589.

Moylan FMB, Seldin EB, Shannon DC, et al: Defective primary dentition in survivors of neonatal mechanical ventilation. *J Pediatr* 1980;96:106.

Perlman J, Thach B: Respiratory origin of fluctuations in arterial blood pressure in premature infants with respiratory distress syndrome. *Pediatrics* 1988;81:399-403.

Sherman JM, Lowitt S, Stephenson C, et al: Factors influencing acquired subglottic stenosis in infants. *J Pediatr* 1986;109:322.

Simbruner G, Coradello H, Fodor M, et al: Effect of tracheal suction on oxygenation, circulation, and lung mechanics in newborn infants. *Arch Dis Child* 1981;56:326.

Tarnow-Mordi W: Is routine endotracheal suction justified? *Arch Dis Child* 1991;66:374-375.

Wimberley PD, Lou HC, Pedersen H, et al: Hypertensive peaks in the pathogenesis of intraventricular hemorrhage in the newborn. Abolition by phenobarbitone sedation. *Acta Paediatr Scand* 1982;71:537-542.

Wung JT, Driscoll JM, Epstein RA, et al: A new device for CPAP by nasal route. *Crit Care Med* 1975;3:76.

Surfactant Administration

Bloom BT, Delmore P, Kattwinkel J: Surfactant prophylaxis increases costs at > 30 weeks. *Pediatr Res* 1994;35:1286A.

Lendig JW, Notter RH, Cox C, et al: A comparison of surfactant as immediate prophylaxis and as rescue therapy in newborns of less than 30 weeks' gestation. *N Engl J Med* 1991;324:865-871.

Segerer H, Van Gelder W, Angenent FWM, et al: Pulmonary distribution and efficacy of exogenous surfactant in lung-lavaged rabbits are influenced by the instillation technique. *Pediatr Res* 1993;34:490-494.

Sitler CG, Turnage CS, McFadden BE, et al: Pump administration of exogenous surfactant: effects on oxygenation, heart rate, and chest wall movement of premature infants. *J Perinatol* 1993;13:197.

Soll RF, McQueen MC: *Respiratory Distress Syndrome in Effective Care of the Newborn Infant.* Oxford University Press, 1992, pp 325-355.

Survanta® package insert. Columbus, Ohio: Ross Laboratories Division of Abbott Laboratories, June 1991.

Ueda T, Ikegami M, Rider ED, et al: Distribution of surfactant and ventilation in surfactant-treated preterm lambs. *J Appl Physiol* 1994;76:45-55.

Zola EM, Gunkel JH, Chan RK, et al: Comparison of three dosing procedures for administration of bovine surfactant to neonates with respiratory distress syndrome. *J Pediatr* 1993;122:453-459.

Positive Pressure Ventilatory Support

Bhutani VK, Abbasi S, Sivieri EM: Continuous skeletal muscle paralysis: effect on neonatal pulmonary mechanics. *Pediatrics* 1988;81:419.

Bland RD, Kim MH, Light MJ, et al: High frequency mechanical ventilation in severe hyaline membrane disease. An alternative treatment? *Crit Care Med* 1980;8:275-280.

Boros SJ, Matalon SV, Ewald R, et al: The effect of independent variations in inspiratory-expiratory ratio and end expiratory pressure during mechanical ventilation in hyaline membrane disease: the significance of mean airway pressure. *J Pediatr* 1977;91:794.

Chan V, Greenough A: Inspiratory and expiratory times for infants ventilator-dependent beyond the first week. *Acta Paediatr* 1994;83:1022.

Chatburn RL: Physiologic and methodologic issues regarding humidity therapy. *J Pediatr* 1989;114:416-420.

Crone RK, Favorito J: The effects of pancuronium bromide on infants with hyaline membrane disease. *J Pediatr* 1980;97:991.

Drew JH: Immediate intubation at birth of the very-low-birth-weight infant. *Am J Dis Child* 1982;136:207-210.

Edberg KE, Sandberg K, Silberberg A, et al: Lung volume, gas mixing, and mechanics of breathing in mechanically ventilated very low birth weight infants with idiopathic respiratory distress syndrome. *Pediatr Res* 1991; 30:496-500.

Enhorning G, Holm BA: Disruption of pulmonary surfactant's ability to maintain openness of a narrow tube. *J Appl Physiol* 1993;74:2922-2927.

Feihl F, Perret C: Permissive hypercapnia. How permissive should we be? *Am J Respir Crit Care Med* 1994;150:1722-1737.

Finer NN, Tomney PM: Controlled evaluation of muscle relaxation in the ventilated neonate. *Pediatrics* 1981;67:641.

Hansen TN, Corbet AJS, Kenny JD, et al: Effects of oxygen and constant positive pressure breathing on aADCO$_2$ in hyaline membrane disease. *Pediatr Res* 1979;13:1167.

Hansen TN, Corbet AJS: Principles of respiratory monitoring and therapy. In: Ballard R, Taeusch W, eds. *Schaffer's Diseases of the Newborn.* WB Saunders, 1991, pp 488-498.

Hanssler L, Tennhoff W, Roll C: Membrane humidification - a new method for humidification of respiratory gases in ventilator treatment of neonates. *Arch Dis Child* 1992;67:1182-1184.

Heicher DA, Kasting DS, Harrod JR: Prospective clinical comparison of two methods for mechanical ventilation of neonates: rapid rate and short inspiratory time versus slow rate and long inspiratory time. *J Pediatr* 1981; 98:957.

Henry GW, Stevens DC, Schreiner RL: Respiratory paralysis to improve oxygenation and mortality in large newborn infants with respiratory distress. *J Pediatr Surg* 1979;14:761.

Herman S, Reynolds EOR: Methods for improving oxygenation in infants mechanically ventilated for severe hyaline membrane disease. *Arch Dis Child* 1973;48:612.

John E, Ermocilla R, Golden J, et al: Effects of gas temperature and particulate water on rabbit lungs during ventilation. *Pediatr Res* 1980;14:1186-1191.

Kano S, Lanteri CJ, Pemberton PJ, et al: Fast versus slow ventilation for neonates. *Am Rev Respir Dis* 1993;148:578-584.

Landers S, Hansen TN, Corbet AJS, et al: Optimal constant positive airway pressure assessed by aADCO$_2$ in hyaline membrane disease. *Pediatr Res* 1986;20:884-889.

Lesouef PN, England SJ, Bryan AC: Total resistance of the respiratory system in preterm infants with and without an endotracheal tube. *J Pediatr* 1984;104:108.

Levene MI, Quinn M: Use of sedatives and muscle relaxants in newborn babies receiving mechanical ventilation. *Arch Dis Child* 1992;67:870-873.

Liu M, Wang L, Li E, et al: Pulmonary surfactant will secure free airflow through a narrow tube. *J Appl Physiol* 1991;71:742-748.

Pietsch JB, Nagaraj HS, Groff DB: Necrotizing tracheobronchitis: a new indication for emergency bronchoscopy in the neonate. *J Pediatr Surg* 1985; 20:391.

Pollitzer MJ, Reynolds EOR, Shaw DG: Pancuronium during mechanical ventilation speeds recovery of lungs of infants with hyaline membrane disease. *Lancet* 1981;February:346.

Primhak RA: Factors associated with pulmonary air leak in premature infants receiving mechanical ventilation. *J Pediatr* 1983;102:764.

Richardson P, Pace WR, Valdes E, et al: Time dependence of lung mechanics in preterm lambs. *Pediatr Res* 1992;31:276-279.

Sandberg K, Edberg K-E, Benton W, et al: Surfactant improves gas mixing and alveolar ventilation in preterm lambs. *Pediatr Res* 1991;30:181.

Schreiner MS, Downes JJ, Kettrick RG, et al: Chronic respiratory failure in infants with prolonged ventilator dependency. *JAMA* 1987;258:3398.

Simbruner G: Inadvertent positive end-expiratory pressure in mechanically ventilated newborn infants: detection and effect on lung mechanics and gas exchange. *J Pediatr* 1986;108:589.

Spitzer AR, Fox WW: Postextubation atelectasis - the role of oral versus nasal endotracheal tubes. *J Pediatr* 1982;100:806.

Stewart AR, Finer NN, Peters KL: Effects of alterations of inspiratory and expiratory pressures and inspiratory/expiratory ratios on mean airway pressure, blood gases, and intracranial pressure. *Pediatrics* 1981;67:474.

Tarnow-Mordi WO, Griffiths ERP, Wilkinson AR: Low inspired gas temperature and respiratory complications in very low birth weight infants. *J Pediatr* 1989;114:438-442.

UK Collaborative Collective Trial Group: UK collaborative randomized trial of neonatal ECMO. *Lancet* 1996;348:75-82.

Vilstrup C, Gommers D, Bos JAH, et al: Natural surfactant instilled in premature lambs increases lung volume and improves ventilation homogeneity within five minutes. *Pediatr Res* 1992;32:595-599.

Vilstrup CT, Bjorklund LJ, Larsson A, et al: Functional residual capacity and ventilation homogeneity in mechanically ventilated small neonates. *J Appl Physiol* 1992;73:276-283.

Wung JT, Driscoll JM, Epstein RA, et al: A new device for CPAP by nasal route. *Crit Care Med* 1975;3:76.

Wung JT: Respiratory management for low birth weight infants. *Neonatal Intensive Care* 1994;January/February:32-33.

SIMV

Ahluwalia JS, Morley CJ, Mockridge JNA: Computerized determination of spontaneous inspiratory and expiratory times in premature neonates during intermittent positive pressure ventilation. II: results from 20 babies. *Arch Dis Child* 1994;70:F161-F164.

Bernstein G, Mannino FL, Heldt GP, et al: Randomized multicenter trial comparing synchronized and conventional intermittent mandatory ventilation in neonates. *J Pediatr* 1996;128:453-463.

Bernstein G, Cleary JP, Heldt GP, et al: Response time and reliability of three neonatal patient-triggered ventilators. *Am Rev Respir Dis* 1993;148:358-364.

Bernstein G, Heldt GP, Mannino FL: Increased and more consistent tidal volumes during synchronized intermittent mandatory ventilation in newborn infants. *Am J Respir Crit Care Med* 1994;150:1444-1448.

deBoer RC, Jones A, Ward PS, et al: Long term trigger ventilation in neonatal respiratory distress syndrome. *Arch Dis Child* 1993;68:308-311.

Greenough A, Greenall F: Patient triggered ventilation in premature neonates. *Arch Dis Child* 1988;63:77-78.

Greenough A, Pool J: Neonatal patient triggered ventilation. *Arch Dis Child* 1988;63:394-397.

Hird MF, Greenough A: Randomized trial of patient triggered ventilation versus high frequency positive pressure ventilation in acute respiratory distress. *J Perinat Med* 1991;19:379-384.

Mehta A, Callan K, Wright BM, et al: Patient triggered ventilation in the newborn. *Lancet* 1986;2:18-19.

Rennie JM, South M, Morely CJ: Cerebral blood flow velocity variability in infants receiving assisted ventilation. *Arch Dis Child* 1987;62:1247.

South M, Morely CJ: Synchronous mechanical ventilation of the neonate. *Arch Dis Child* 1986;61:1190-1195.

Truog WE, Jackson JC: Alternative modes of ventilation in the prevention and treatment of bronchopulmonary dysplasia. *Clin Perinatol* 1992;19:621-647.

Visveshwara N, Freeman B, Peck M, et al: Patient-triggered synchronized assisted ventilation of newborns: report of a preliminary study and three years' experience. *J Perinatol* 1991;11:347-354.

High-Frequency Jet Ventilation

Boros SJ, Mammel MD, Coleman JM: Neonatal high-frequency jet ventilation: four years' experience. *Pediatrics* 1985:75:657.

Carlo WA, Beoglos A, Chatburn RL, et al: High-frequency jet ventilation in neonatal pulmonary hypertension. *Am J Dis Child* 1989;143:233.

Carlo WA, Chatburn RL, Martin RJ, et al: Decrease in airway pressure during high-frequency jet ventilation in infants with respiratory distress syndrome. *J Pediatr* 1984;04:101.

Froese AB, Bryan AC: State of the art: high-frequency ventilation. *Am Rev Respir Dis* 1987;135:1363-1374.

Keszler M, Donn SM, Bucciarelli RL, et al: Multicenter controlled trial comparing high-frequency jet ventilation and conventional mechanical ventilation in newborn infants with pulmonary interstitial emphysema. *J Pediatr* 1991;119:85-93.

Mammel MC, Gordon MJ, Connett JE, et al: Comparison of high-frequency jet ventilation and conventional mechanical ventilation in a meconium aspiration model. *J Pediatr* 1983;103:630.

Slutsky AS: Nonconventional methods of ventilation. *Am Rev Respir Dis* 1988;138:175.

Trindade W, Goldberg RN, Bancalari E, et al: Conventional vs high-frequency jet ventilation in a piglet model of meconium aspiration: comparison of pulmonary and hemodynamic effects. *Pediatrics* 1985;107:115.

Wiswell, TE, Graziani LJ, Kornhauser MS, et al: High-frequency jet ventilation in the early management of respiratory distress syndrome is associated with a greater risk for adverse outcomes. *Pediatrics* 1996;98:1035-1043.

High-Frequency Oscillatory Ventilation (HFOV)

Bancalari A, Gerhardt T, Bancalari E, et al: Gas trapping with high-frequency ventilation: jet versus oscillatory ventilation. *J Pediatr* 1987;110:617-622.

Bryan AC, Froese AB: Reflections on the HiFi trial. *Pediatrics* 1991; 87:565-567.

Carter JM, Gerstmann DR, Clark RH, et al: High-frequency oscillatory ventilation and extracorporeal membrane oxygenation for the treatment of acute neonatal respiratory failure. *Pediatrics* 1990;85:159-164.

Clark RH, Dykes FD, Bachman TE, et al: Intraventricular hemorrhage and high-frequency ventilation: a meta-analysis of prospective clinical trials. *Pediatrics* 1996;98:1058-1061.

Clark RH, Gerstmann DR, Null DM, et al: Prospective randomized comparison of high frequency oscillatory and conventional ventilation in respiratory distress syndrome. *Pediatrics* 1992;89:5-12.

Clark RH, Gerstmann DR, Null DM: Pulmonary interstitial emphysema treated by high frequency oscillatory ventilation. *Crit Care Med* 1986; 14:926-930.

Clark RH, Yoder BA, Sell MS: Prospective, randomized comparison of high-frequency oscillation and conventional ventilation in candidates for extracorporeal membrane oxygenation. *J Pediatr* 1994;24:447-454.

Frantz ID, Wethammer J, Stark AR: High-frequency ventilation in premature infants with lung disease: adequate gas exchange at low tracheal pressure. *Pediatrics* 1983;71:483-488.

Frantz ID: High-frequency ventilation. In: *Neonatal Respiratory Diseases.* Associates in Medical Marketing Co., Newtown, PA, 1995;5:1.

Froese AB, Butler PO, Fletcher WA, et al: High-frequency oscillatory ventilation in premature infants with respiratory failure: a preliminary report. *Anesth Analg* 1987;66:814-824.

Gerstmann DR, DeLemos RA, Coalson JJ, et al: Influence of ventilatory technique on pulmonary baro-injury in baboons with hyaline membrane disease. *Pediatr Pulmonol* 1988;5:82-91.

Gerstmann DR, Minton SD, Stoddard RA, et al: The Provo multicenter early-HFOV trial: improved pulmonary and clinical outcomes in respiratory distress syndrome. *Pediatrics* 1996;98:1044-1057.

Hamilton PP, Onayemi A, Smyth JA, et al: Comparison of conventional and high frequency ventilation: oxygenation and lung pathology. *J Appl Physiol* 1983;55:131-138.

HiFi Study Group: High-frequency oscillatory ventilation compared with conventional mechanical ventilation in the treatment of respiratory failure in preterm infants. *N Engl J Med* 1989;320:88-93.

HiFO Study Group. Randomized study of high-frequency oscillatory ventilation in infants with severe respiratory distress syndrome. *J Pediatr* 1993; 122:609-619.

Marchak BE, Thompson WK, Duffty P, et al: Treatment of RDS by high-frequency oscillatory ventilation: a preliminary report. *J Pediatr* 1981; 99:287-292.

Ogawa Y, Miyasaka K, Kawano T, et al: A multicenter randomized trial of high-frequency oscillatory ventilation as compared with conventional mechanical ventilation in preterm infants with respiratory failure. *Early Hum Dev* 1993;32:1-10.

Slutsky AS: Nonconventional methods of ventilation. *Am Rev Respir Dis* 1988;138:175.

ECMO

Bartlett RH, Roloff DW, Cornell RG, et al: Extracorporeal circulation in neonatal respiratory failure: a prospective randomized study. *J Pediatr* 1985; 76:479.

Campbell LR, Bunyapen C, Holmes GL, et al: Right common carotid artery ligation in extracorporeal membrane oxygenation. *J Pediatr* 1988; 113:110.

Cilley RE, Zwischenberger JB, Andrews AF, et al: Intracranial hemorrhage during extracorporeal membrane oxygenation in neonates. *J Pediatr* 1986;78:699.

Cornish JD, Heiss KF, Clark RH, et al: Efficacy of venovenous extracorporeal membrane oxygenation for neonates with respiratory and circulatory compromise. *J Pediatr* 1993;122:105-109.

Hirschl RB, Schumacher RE, Snedecor SN, et al: The efficacy of extracorporeal life support in premature and low birth weight newborns. *J Pediatr Surg* 1993;28:1336-1341.

Hocker JR, Simpson PM, Rabalais GP, et al: Extracorporeal membrane oxygenation and early-onset group B streptococcal sepsis. *Pediatrics* 1992; 89:1-4.

Hofkosh D, Thompson AE, Nozza RJ, et al: Ten years of extracorporeal membrane oxygenation: neurodevelopmental outcome. *Pediatrics* 1991; 87:549-555.

Kanto WP: A decade of experience with neonatal extracorporeal membrane oxygenation. *J Pediatr* 1994;124:335-347.

Ogawa Y, Miyasaka K, Kawano T, et al: A multicenter randomized trial of high-frequency oscillatory ventilation as compared with conventional mechanical ventilation in preterm infants with respiratory failure. *Early Hum Dev* 1993;32:1-10.

O'Rourke PP, Crone RK, Vacanti JP, et al: Extracorporeal membrane oxygenation and conventional medical therapy in neonates with persistent pulmonary hypertension of the newborn: a prospective randomized study. *Pediatrics* 1989;84:957-963.

O'Rourke PP, Lillehei CW, Crone RK, et al: The effect of extracorporeal membrane oxygenation on the survival of neonates with high-risk congenital diaphragmatic hernia: 45 cases from a single institution. *J Pediatr Surg* 1991;36:147-152.

Ortega M, Ramos AD, Platzker ACG, et al: Early prediction of ultimate outcome in newborn infants with severe respiratory failure. *J Pediatr* 1988; 113:744.

Wildin SR, Landry SH, Zwischenberger JB: Prospective, controlled study of developmental outcome in survivors of extracorporeal membrane oxygenation: the first 24 months. *Pediatrics* 1994;93:404-408.

Nitric Oxide

Donn SM: Alternatives to ECMO. *Arch Dis Child* 1994;70:F81-F83.

Edwards AD: The pharmacology of inhaled nitric oxide. *Arch Dis Child* 1995;72:F127-F130.

Finer NN, Etches PC, Kamstra B, et al: Inhaled nitric oxide in infants referred for extracorporeal membrane oxygenation: dose response. *J Pediatr* 1993;124:302-307.

Karamanoukian HL, Glick PL, Wilcox DT, et al: Pathophysiology of congenital diaphragmatic hernia. VIII. Inhaled nitric oxide requires exogenous surfactant therapy in the lamb model of congenital diaphragmatic hernia. *J Pediatr Surg* 1995;30:1-4.

Kinsella JP, Ivy DD, Abman SH: Inhaled nitric oxide improves gas exchange and lowers pulmonary vascular resistance in severe experimental hyaline membrane disease. *Pediatr Res* 1994;36:402-408.

Kinsella JP, McQueston JA, Rosenberg AA, et al: Hemodynamic effects of exogenous nitric oxide in ovine transitional pulmonary circulation. *Am J Physiol* 1992;263:H875-H880.

Kinsella JP, McQueston JA, Rosenberg AA, et al: Hemodynamic effects of exogenous nitric oxide in ovine transitional pulmonary circulation. *Am J Physiol* 1992;875-880.

Kinsella JP, Neish SR, Shaffer E, et al: Low-dose inhalational nitric oxide in persistent pulmonary hypertension of the newborn. *Lancet* 1992; 340:819-820.

Kinsella JP, Truog WE, Walsh WF, et al: Randomized, multicenter trial of inhaled nitric oxide and high-frequency oscillatory ventilation in severe, persistent pulmonary hypertension of the newborn. *J Pediatr* 1997;131:55-62.

Roberts JD Jr, Fineman JR, Morin FC III, et al: Inhaled nitric oxide and persistent pulmonary hypertension of the newborn. The Inhaled Nitric Oxide Study Group. *N Engl J Med* 1997;336:605-610.

Roberts JD, Polaner DM, Lang P, et al: Inhaled nitric oxide in persistent pulmonary hypertension of the newborn. *Lancet* 1992;340:818-819.

Shah N, Jacob T, Exler R, et al: Inhaled nitric oxide in congenital diaphragmatic hernia. *J Pediatr Surg* 1994;29:1010-1015.

Walker MW, Kinter MT, Roberts RJ, et al: Nitric oxide-induced cytotoxicity: involvement of cellular resistance to oxidative stress and the role of glutathione in protection. *Pediatr Res* 1995;37:41-49.

Zayek M, Cleveland D, Morin FC: Treatment of persistent pulmonary hypertension in the newborn lamb by inhaled nitric oxide. *J Pediatr* 1993; 122:743-750.

Chapter 11

Nutritional and Gastrointestinal Support for the Infant With Respiratory Distress

Nutritional Support

Nutrition is integral in the management of the infant with respiratory distress. Malnutrition affects respiratory function by impairment of cellular reactions, protective antioxidant mechanisms, immune defenses, and lung development. In addition, *excessive* carbohydrate administration may impair lung function. Consequently, the ability to wean an infant with compromised lung function from ventilatory support may be prolonged without attention to nutritional well-being.

To achieve rates of nutrient accretion (Table 1) similar to those of the fetus, optimal acute and chronic nutrition for high-risk neonates must be maintained. In providing this nutritional support, the clinician must consider the neonate's limited body stores, increased energy expenditure, and potential nutrient-therapy interactions. The goal of nutritional support is to enable a body-weight gain of approximately 15 g/kg/d or, for neonates greater than 35 weeks' gestation, approximately 20 g/d.

This section focuses on the guidelines for the acute and chronic nutritional management of high-risk neonates, most of whom require respiratory support. This population includes the very-low-birth-weight infant (<1,500 g) and the larger, more mature infant with bronchopulmonary dysplasia (BPD).

Parenteral Nutrition

Immaturity or severe illness usually requires that total parenteral nutrition (TPN) is used as the initial mode of nutrition for the high-risk neonate. This support provides intravenous glucose, synthetic amino acids, electrolytes, vitamins, and lipids.

If begun within the first 3 days after birth, glucose plus amino acids has been shown to reverse negative nitrogen balance, increase protein synthesis rate, and elevate the serum concentrations of *essential* amino acids better than solutions containing only glucose. The amino acid solution containing the greatest percentage of essential amino acids (52%) is currently Trophamine® (McGaw, Inc, Irvine, CA). This mixture also appears to improve the solubility of calcium and phosphorus.

Inadequate intakes of calcium and phosphorus can lead to undermineralized bone, rickets, and fractures. Consequently, parenteral solutions must maintain good solubility and delivery of these minerals. Careful attention to factors influencing the solubility of calcium and phosphorus (eg, pH, temperature, calcium and phosphorus concentration, and amino acid source and concentration) is a priority.

It is controversial whether the amino acid cysteine (supplemented as hydrochloride, 30 to 40 mg/g amino acids) is essential for high-risk neonates; nonetheless, addition of this amino acid lowers the pH, favoring the solubility of calcium and phosphorus. Occasionally, this results in a mild metabolic acidosis, which is treated with sodium or potassium acetate (1 to 3 mEq/dL); the use of sodium bicarbonate must be avoided in TPN solutions. Finally, to optimize solubility while the solution is mixed, phosphorus should be added before calcium.

Inadequate provision of essential fatty acids may affect growth, produce essential fatty acid deficiency, and hinder the production of pulmonary surfactants. Contem-

Table 1: Suggested Nutrient Intakes for Both Enteral and Parenteral Support*

Nutrient	Enteral per kg/d	Parenteral per kg/d
Energy (kcal)	120	80-90
Protein (g) [†]	3.0-3.8	3.0-3.6
Vitamins		
A (IU) [‡]	700-1,500	700-1,500
D (IU)	400	160
E (IU) [§]	6-25	3.5-7.0
K (µg)	8-10	8-10
B_1 (µg)	110-240	200-350
B_2 (µg)	250-360	150-200
B_6 (µg)	150-210	150-200
B_{12} (µg)	0.3	0.3
Niacin (mg)	3.6-4.8	4.0-6.8
Folic Acid (µg)	25-50	56
Electrolytes [‖]		
Sodium (mEq)	2.0-3.0	2.0-3.0
Potassium (mEq)	2.0-3.0	2.0-3.0
Chloride (mEq)	2.0-3.0	2.0-3.0
Minerals		
Calcium (mg)	120-230	65-104
Phosphorus (mg)	60-140	60-81
Magnesium (mg)	7.9-15.0	4.3-7.2

porary lipid infusions contain 10% (1.1 kcal/mL) or 20% lipid (2.0 kcal/mL) in blends of soy and safflower oils (predominantly as the essential fatty acids: linoleic and linolenic acids). A 20% lipid emulsion, infused throughout a 24-hour period, produces lower serum triglycerides than a 10% emulsion, despite similar lipid intakes.

When TPN is begun during the first 3 days after birth, the composition remains the same, although delivered at a lower

Nutrient	Enteral per kg/d	Parenteral per kg/d
Trace elements		
Iron (mg)[¶]	2.0-6.0	—
Zinc (μg)[#]	1,000	400
Copper (μg)	120-230	20
Selenium (μg)	1.3-3.0	1.5-2.0

* Note: Estimated guidelines for infants <35 weeks' gestation. Consult RDAs for infants >35 weeks' gestation.

† Protein needs can be elevated because of excess losses (chest tubes, ventricular taps, ostomy sites, surgical wounds, PDA ligations) or therapies (corticosteroids).

‡ Vitamin A needs may be greater with increased polyunsaturated fat use and therapy.

§ Vitamin E needs may be greater with increased polyunsaturated fat use and therapy.

‖ Electrolyte needs can be elevated because of losses (ostomy sites, urine, diuretic therapy).

¶ Iron supplementation should begin after 1 month of age.

Zinc needs may be elevated in infants with NEC or those with increased losses or on unfortified human milk.

volume (generally 80 to 100 mL/kg/d). Twenty percent intralipid emulsion is usually initiated no later than the fifth day after birth at 5 mL/kg/d (1 g/kg/d) and advanced by increments of 5 to 10 mL/kg/d (1 to 2 g/kg/d), with a goal of 20 mL/kg/d (4 g/kg/d). Infants on extracorporeal membrane oxygenation (ECMO) may require a separate IV for lipids, since lipids may cause cracked hubs when infused through the ECMO circuit.

Table 2: Energy Distribution from Total Parenteral Nutrition

	TPN each 100 cc	TPN (@ 130 mL/kg)	TPN (@ 130 mL/kg) plus 20% IL (20 mL/kg)
Total calories (kcal)	51.3	66.7	106.7
Glucose 12.5%			
(kcal)	42.5	55.3	55.3
(% calories)	83%	83%	52%
Amino acids			
(kcal)	8.8	11.4	11.4
(% calories)	17%	17%	11%
Intralipid 20%			
(kcal)	—	—	40
(% calories)	0%	0%	37%

Peripheral TPN solutions of 12.5% glucose and 2.2% amino acids infused at 130 mL/kg/d, when coadministered with IV lipid at 4 g/kg/d (20 mL/kg/d), provide a balanced distribution of calories and optimal weight gain (Tables 2 and 3). The quantity of protein, however, may be increased (up to 4 g/kg/d) during times of increased losses or increased nitrogen demands, such as those following necrotizing enterocolitis (NEC) or gastrointestinal surgery.

The distribution of fat and lipid calories is important and should parallel that in enteral nutrition—approximately 45% to 50% glucose, 40% to 50% lipid, and 10% to 15% protein. There are 3.4 kcal/g in glucose, 9 kcal/g in lipid, and 4 kcal/g in amino acid. High glucose-containing TPN solutions (glucose providing more than 50% of calories or >12 mg/kg/min) may increase carbon dioxide production and raise the P_{CO_2}.

Nursery guidelines for TPN should specify biochemical monitoring to avoid toxicity or deficiencies (Table 4). These should include protein and calorie status (albumin and blood urea nitrogen [BUN]), and renal (BUN, creatinine, and electrolytes), bone (calcium, magnesium, phosphorus, and alkaline phosphatase), and liver function tests (fractionated bilirubins, alanine transaminase [ALT], and gamma glutaryl transferase [GGT]).

Enteral Nutrition

Enteral nutrition should be initiated as soon as clinical stability allows. The TPN-associated risks of cholestatic jaundice, undermineralized bone, and infections are lessened with enteral feeding. Small volumes of 'trophic' milk feedings (10 to 20 mL/kg/d) can safely be initiated in most infants once physiologic stability in the infant is achieved—as early as the first week after birth—even in conjunction with mechanical ventilation or indwelling umbilical catheters. For the high-risk neonate, enteral nutrition has been shown to stimulate gastrointestinal trophic hormones, motor activity, and intestinal development and to improve feeding tolerance, growth, and biochemical markers of nutritional status. As the infant matures and feeding tolerance improves, the volume is advanced in increments of 10 to 20 mL/kg/d to achieve full enteral feeding of 150 mL/kg/d. As milk volume increases, the TPN fluids are diminished accordingly.

Methods of enteral feeding. Milk is administered via orogastric, nasogastric, or transpyloric feeding tubes until the infant is sufficiently mature to coordinate sucking, swallowing, and breathing. There are advantages and disadvantages to each tube-feeding method (Table 5). When compared with the transpyloric method, gastric feedings result in increased fat absorption (through stimulation of gastric lipase), increased potassium absorption, decreased risk of bacterial overgrowth and intestinal perforation, and decreased need for radiographic verification of tube position.

Table 3: Neonatal Parenteral Nutrition

	per 100 mL	per 130 mL/kg/d
Glucose (g)	12.5	16.25
Amino acids (g)	2.2	2.9
NaCl (mEq)	2.6	3.4
Ca gluconate (mEq)*	2.5-4.0	3.25-5.2
Ca gluconate (mg Ca)*	50-80	65-104
$MgSO_4$ (mEq)	0.5	0.65
$MgSO_4$ (mg)	6.0	7.8
K_2PO_4 (mmol P)*	1.5-2.0	1.95-2.6
K_2PO_4 (mg P)*	46-62	60-81
K_2PO_4 (mEq K)*	2.2-2.9	2.9-3.8
KCl (mEq)	0.2-0	0.26-0
Total K (mEq)	(2.4-2.9)	(3.1-3.8)
Cysteine HCl	30 mg/g amino acids	30 mg/g amino acids

Vitamins will be added daily as 40% of a vial of MVI®
Pediatric (per kg) for infants <2.5 kg, and 1 vial
   for infants >2.5 kg.
Heparin is added to a concentration of 1 U/mL.
10% Intralipid (54% linoleic acid), 1.1 kcal/mL
20% Intralipid (50% linoleic acid), 2.0 kcal/mL

*Note: use the lower Ca and P concentration initially;
   for TPN after 2 weeks, use higher concentrations.

Transpyloric feedings are used in infants who have failed the orogastric method, usually because of dysmotility and poor gastric emptying. This method may decrease the risk of milk aspiration.

Milk may be infused either continuously or intermittently (every 2 to 4 hours). The continuous method may be better tolerated in infants weighing less than 1,500 g, because less volume is delivered per feeding, which may benefit compliance. Compared with intermittent feeding, the continu-

Contents of 1 Vial (5 mL) of MVI-Pediatric

Vitamin A	2300 IU (690 µg)	Thiamin (B_1)	1.2 mg
Vitamin D	400 IU (10 µg)	Riboflavin (B_2)	1.4 mg
		Niacin	17 mg
Vitamin E	7 IU (7 mg)	Pyridoxine (B_6)	1.0 mg
		Folic Acid	140 µg
Vitamin K	200 µg	Vitamin B_{12}	1.0 µg
Vitamin C	80 mg		
Pantothenic acid	5 mg		
Biotin	20 µg		

Daily Trace Element Requirements

Trace elements (µg/kg/d):	<2.5 kg	>2.5 kg
Zinc	300	100
Copper	40	10
Chromium	0.4	0.1
Manganese	10	2.5
Selenium	2	1.5
mL/kg/d	1.0	0.1

ous infusion method results in lower energy expenditure, greater nutrient absorption, and improved pulmonary function. Because of these advantages, neonates with chronic cardiopulmonary and gastrointestinal disorders particularly may benefit from the continuous infusion method.

Intermittent or bolus tube feeding provides direct delivery of milk under the nurse's observation every few hours. This practice allows less time for milk fat, calcium, and zinc to separate out or adhere to tubing and less time for the

Table 4: Labs–Infants on TPN *Exclusively*

	Initially	Short-term	Long-term
Urine glucose	q void	q.d.	q.d.
Triglyceride	4 hours after each change in infusion rate, then (depending if jaundice, SGA*, septic, or severe cardiopulmonary disease):		
	q.o.d.	twice weekly	q wk
Lytes, glucose	q.d.	twice weekly	q wk
BUN, creatinine	q.d.	twice weekly	q wk then q o wk
Calcium	∅	q wk	q o wk
Mg, PO₄, and Alk Phos	∅	q wk	q o wk
Albumin (and prealbumin)	∅	q wk	q o wk
Bilirubin U/C, ALT, GGT	∅	q o wk	q o wk

*SGA = small for gestational age

milk to interact with medications. Gastrointestinal hormonal stimulation and glucose tolerance have been shown to be more physiologic when the intermittent feeding method is used.

Generally, for neonates less than 1,500 g, we initiate feedings with the continuous orogastric infusion method to optimize delivery of the milk. We use an automated infusion pump with an attached syringe pointed upward against gravity to avoid loss of fat. The syringes hold 3 to 4 hours of milk

Table 5: Methods for Providing Enteral Nutrients

	Orogastric	Transpyloric	Gastrostomy
Possible uses	Prematurity and short-term feeding problems;	Slow gastric empytying	Long-term feeding problems
	30-day tubes available	Severe GER	
Routine care	Size 5 or 8 French tube	Difficult to place	Foley catheter
	Change q feed or q day	Change q 3 days	Change monthly/ p.r.n.
	Infusion by gravity	Infusion by gravity	Infusion by gravity
	Liquids only	Liquids only	Liquids, cereal, and pureed solids
Complications	Aspiration	Poor fat absorption	Skin irritation
	Vagal episodes	Intestinal perforation	Granulation tissue
	GI irritation or bleeding	Renal perforation	*Staphylococcus* cellulitis

and are changed every 6 to 8 hours. Once the infant achieves complete enteral feedings and body weight is greater than 1,500 g, the feeding method is changed to intermittent, three-hourly feedings. As the infant achieves physiologic stability, non-nutritive feeding and skin-to-skin contact between the

Table 6: Nutrient Composition of Mature Human Milk, Fortified Human Milk, Preterm Formulas, and Full-Term Infant Formulas

	HM	FHM (MJ)	SSC-24 (R)
Energy			
(kcal/oz)	15-24	18-26	24
(kcal/dL)	50-80	60-90	81
Protein			
(g/dL)	1.0	1.7	2.2
(% whey/% casein)	70/30	70/30	60/40
(% total calories)	6	9	11
Fat			
(g/dL)	3.5	3.5	4.4
(% MCT/% LCT)	2/98	2/98	50/50
(% total calories)	52	41	47
Carbohydrate			
(g/dL)	7.0	9.7	8.5
% lactose/% polymers	100/0	78/22	50/50
(% total calories)	42	50	42
Calcium (mg/dL)	26	116	145
Phosphorus (mg/dL)	14	59	73
Sodium (mg/dL)	20	27	35
Potassium (mg/dL)	60	76	104
Zinc (mg/dL)	0.32	1.00	1.2
Iron (mg/dL) (in iron fortified formulations)	<0.1	<0.1	1.5
Vitamin A (IU/dL)	500	1,350	544
Vitamin D (IU/dL)	<10	210	120
Renal solute (mOsm/dL)	7.0	—	15.0
Osmolarity (mOsm/dL)	260	380	270

HM = Approximate values for mature human milk;
FHM = Fortified HM with 4 packets of Enfamil Human Milk Fortifier (MJ) per 100 mL HM;
SSC = Similac Special Care;
EPF = Enfamil Premature formula:

EPF-24 (MJ)	SIM-24 (R)	ENF-24 (MJ)	SIM-20 (R)	ENF-20 (MJ)
24	24	24	20	20
81	81	81	67	67
2.4	2.2	1.7	1.4	1.4
60/40	18/82	60/40	18/82	60/40
12	11	9	8	8
4.0	4.3	4.2	3.6	3.5
40/60	4/96	8/92	8/92	4/96
44	47	47	48	48
8.9	8.5	8.7	7.2	7.3
40/60	100/0	100/0	100/0	100/0
44	42	44	43	43
131	73	62	49	52
67	57	42	37	35
31	27	21	19	18
82	107	86	73	72
1.2	0.6	0.8	0.5	0.5
1.4	1.4	1.4	1.2	1.2
992	240	238	200	206
214	48	48	40	42
15.0	14.6	11.7	10.0	9.8
260	340	320	270	270

SIM = Similac;
ENF = Enfamil;
MJ = Mead Johnson, a Bristol-Myers Squibb Co, Evansville, Ind;
R = Ross Products Div., Abbott Laboratories, Columbus, Ohio;

parent and infant are introduced, to prepare the infant to learn to feed orally. Oral feeding generally is introduced after 32 weeks' postmenstrual age but more often is not completely achieved until 35 weeks. Infants greater than 35 weeks and 2,000 g body weight can usually tolerate initially ordering all feedings orally.

Human milk. Human milk is the most frequent choice of feeding in most nurseries. Data are emerging to suggest that human milk improves nutrient absorption, stimulates gastrointestinal function, and benefits host defense. The protein composition is whey dominant (70% whey, 30% casein) (Table 6). The whey-protein fraction tends to be more soluble and more easily digested compared with casein, and it contains the host-defense proteins: lactoferrin, secretory IgA, and lysozyme. During the initial 2 to 4 weeks of lactation, preterm milk usually has a greater protein content than term milk but this declines during lactation. Therefore, optimal intakes of protein may be a concern after the first 2 weeks of feeding.

Fat absorption from human milk generally is excellent because of the presence of human milk lipase and the unique packaging of fatty acids in the fat globule (the particular fatty acids' arrangement on the glycerol backbone improves their availability for enzymatic cleavage). The presence of cholesterol is important for membrane stability. Very-long-chain polyunsaturated fatty acids (eg, docosahexaenoic acid [DHA], and arachidonic acid), which are present in human milk, but not bovine milk, are membrane constituents with a predilection for retinal membranes. Red blood cell concentrations of DHA, for example, remain elevated in infants fed human milk, but decline rapidly with formula feeding. In low-birth-weight (LBW) infants <1,500 g, an important association is seen between increased dietary DHA and improved visual acuity and visual evoked responses.

The concentration of fat in human milk rises during a single milk expression. The higher-fat-containing hind milk often is used in high-risk infants to provide a greater energy intake and to promote weight gain. Mothers can be taught to fractionate their milk collection and bring only the hind milk to the nursery. (Mothers discard the first 2 to 3 minutes of milk that is expressed from each breast. The subsequently expressed milk is hind milk.)

Mineral absorption from human milk is high, but the quantity of calcium, phosphorus, and sodium is inadequate to meet the greater needs of the LBW (<2,500 g) infant, the infant who has chronically received TPN, or the infant who requires restricted fluid intake. For this reason, a multicomponent fortifier containing energy, protein, calcium, phosphorus, sodium, and multivitamins should be added to the milk (Table 6). It is not uncommon for infants to require 160 to 200 mL/kg/d of fortified human milk. Human milk fortification continues until the infant reaches 2,000 g body weight and 35 weeks' postmenstrual age or until the infant achieves successful full oral feeding.

Optimizing nutrition with human milk fortifiers is important because human milk may have profound benefits for the high-risk infant's gastrointestinal function and host defense. A variety of proteins, peptides, hormones, and specific growth factors are responsible for better feeding tolerance and gastric emptying than that of formula-fed infants.

Commercial formulas. Several state-of-the-art enteral formulas are designed specifically for the high-risk neonate to avoid nutrient deficits and to compensate for the effects of immature intestinal function (Table 6). Both the quantity and quality of the nutrients are increased to match the high rate of fetal nutrient accretion. All products contain protein exceeding 3 g/kg/d. Most formulas have a whey:casein ratio of 60:40. Approximately 50% of the long-chain fats are replaced by medium-chain fatty acids. The lactose content is reduced to approximately 50% by the addition of glucose polymers to lessen the osmolality and because of the premature infant's immature lactase activity. All preterm formulas contain abundant calcium and phosphorus and an appropriate osmolality and renal solute load.

Recognizing the nutritional quantity and quality differences among formulas for preterm and those for full-term infants is important. The latter contain significantly lower quantities of protein, calcium, phosphorus, vitamins, and trace elements. Soy-based formulas are not recommended for LBW infants because of poor protein quality and diminished mineral absorption. The hydrolysate-based formulas also have low levels of many nutrients and generally are derived solely from casein. Casein contains more aromatic and sulfur-containing amino acids, which are more difficult for the LBW infant to metabolize.

To achieve adequate weight gain, 150 to 160 mL/kg/d is generally needed. Initially, the preterm formulas are administered in small volumes of 10 to 20 mL/kg/d at half strength. The concentration is changed to full strength, and, subsequently, the volume is increased by stepwise increments of 10 to 20 mL/kg/d.

Micronutrient Supplementation

Along with macronutrients (calories and protein), supplementation of micronutrients (vitamins, minerals, and trace elements) may be necessary (Table 7) to provide an adequate intake and weight gain.

Infants on 150 to 160 mL/kg/d fortified human milk (FHM), Similac® Special Care (SSC), or Enfamil® Premature Formula (EPF) generally receive adequate amounts of calories, protein, vitamins, and trace elements (FHM-fed infants may require 180 to 200 mL/kg/d).

Iron can be provided using Fer-In-Sol® (Mead Johnson Nutritionals, a Bristol-Myers Squibb Co, Evansville, Ind) at 2 mg/kg/d elemental iron for infants on FHM by 1 month of age. At these ages, SSC or EPF with iron should be used. This provides 2 mg/kg/d of elemental iron when given at 150 mL/kg/d.

Table 7: Enteral Dietary Supplements

Additive	Caloric content	Source
Glucose	3.4 kcal/g	dextrose
Polycose powder (R)	3.8 kcal/g	glucose polymers
Polycose liquid (R)	2.0 kcal/mL	glucose polymers
Corn oil	8.4 kcal/mL	LCT (34% EFA)
MCT oil (MJ)	7.7 kcal/mL	MCT (0% EFA)
Microlipid (S)	4.5 kcal/mL	LCT (74% EFA)
Casec (MJ)	0.88 g protein/g	calcium caseinate
ProMod (R)	0.76 g protein/g	whey protein concentrate
Multivitamins*	1 mL/d if 20 kcal formula @ <1 L/d	
Multivitamins with fluoride (.25 mg Fl/mL)	1 mL/d if human milk @ <1 L/d	
Iron drops**	2 mg/kg/d elemental iron	

MCT—Medium-chain triglycerides; LCT—Long-chain triglycerides; EFA—Essential fatty acids; R=Ross; MJ=Mead Johnson

*Vi-Daylin® (Ross Products Div., Abbott Laboratories, Columbus, Ohio), Poly-Vi-Sol (Mead Johnson); **Fer-In-Sol (Mead Johnson), 25 mg/mL elemental iron as ferrous sulfur with vitamin C.

Once infants are >35 postmenstrual weeks, are >2 kg, and are orally consuming 180 mL/kg/d, then using 20 kcal/oz standard formulas with iron or unfortified human milk is appropriate. However, until the infant ingests a quart per day of standard formula or human milk, a multivitamin supplement is suggested (Table 7).

Nutritional Assessment

Laboratory values and growth goals should be established and then routinely monitored when caring for high-risk neonates. Laboratory values used to monitor enteral nutrition include: albumin, calcium, phosphorus, and alkaline phosphatase (initially every week, then every other week if feeding and clinical status have been stable) (Table 8). Monitoring prealbumin or BUN is helpful if assessment of acute changes in nutritional or clinical status is needed.

Finally, the high-risk infant should achieve an average weight gain of 15 g/kg/d during a week (or 20 g/d for the mature, >35 weeks' gestation infant), head circumference gain of 1.0 cm per week, and serial increases in body or knee-to-heel length.

Chronic Nutritional Management

Chronic nutritional management is especially important in infants with BPD who are often fluid restricted and receiving diuretics. Furthermore, the infant with BPD has increased energy expenditure and nutrient needs. With volume limitations of 100 to 130 mL/kg/d and increased metabolic demands, growth is often poor.

Calorie and protein supplements are available for addition to the infant's milk (Table 7). Caution is advised with this practice. Nutrient ratios (Table 9) can easily be altered inappropriately. Routine supplementation with glucose polymers, for example, can increase the carbohydrate load and can potentially increase the infant's respiratory

Table 8: Nutritional Assessment of the High-Risk Neonate

Growth

Body weight gain	Plot on growth grid	daily
Rate of weight gain	15 g/kg/d or 20 g/d	weekly
Length	1 cm/wk	weekly
Head circumference	1 cm/wk	weekly

Biochemical

Protein status	albumin	q o wk
	BUN	q o wk
	prealbumin	as needed
Mineral status	Ca, P, Alk Phos	q o wk
Anemia	Hemoglobin	weekly
	Reticulocyte count	weekly
Cholestasis	Fract. bilirubin	>1 month on
	ALT, GGT	TPN
Poor growth with good intake	zinc	as needed
	Vitamin A	

quotient or cause lactic acidosis. Protein and other minerals important for linear skeletal growth can become diluted. For these reasons, a ready-made, 27 kcal/oz formula may be more appropriate to provide recommended nutrients without the worry of nutrient dilution or additive complications. Mixing powder or concentrate with less water than usual can achieve similar results. In infants with se-

Table 9: Concentrating Infant Formula to 27 Calories/Oz

	Standard 27	20 kcal + Oil	20 kcal + Polycose
Energy	90 kcal/dL	90 kcal/dL	90 kcal/dL
Fat	4.8 g/dL 48% total cal	6.6 g/dL 65% total cal	3.6 g/dL 36% total cal
Carbo-hydrate	9.5 g/dL 42% total cal	6.7 g/dL 30% total cal	14.9 g/dL 66% total cal
Protein	2.5 g/dL 11% total cal	1.4 g/dL 6% total cal	1.4 g/dL 6% total cal

Note that the percentage calories from protein is increased by concentrating a standard formula to 27 kcal/oz compared with adding additional calories as fat or carbohydrate. The distribution of calories is imbalanced by adding only fat or carbohydrate.

vere BPD who are over 6 months of age, selected formulas (30 kcal/oz) may be considered (see *BPD*, Chapter 5). Solid foods using iron-enriched cereal and vitamin A-rich foods should also begin with 1 to 2 tsp/d, to encourage development of oral motor skills.

Besides the usual parameters (Table 8), nutritional assessment should include the evaluation of fluid and electrolyte balance. Renal ultrasounds to rule out nephrocalcinosis, and wrist radiographs to evaluate the possibility of rickets, may also be warranted in some infants. Finally, growth goals should include chronologic and corrected age comparisons on the National Center for Health Statistics' growth charts.

By Christina J. Valentine, RD, Richard J. Schanler, MD, and Stephen A. Abrams, MD

Table 10: Commonly Used GI Medications

	Drug	Dose
Antacids and H$_2$ blockers	Aluminum hydroxide	0.5 to 1.0 mL/dose PO q 1 to 2 hours
	Aluminum hydroxide with magnesium hydroxide	0.5 to 1.0 mL/dose PO q 1 to 2 hours
	Ranitidine hydrochloride	1.5-2.0 mg/kg/dose q 6-12 hours PO
		1.5 mg/kg dose q 6 hours IV
	Cimetidine hydrochloride	2.5-5 mg/kg/dose q 6 hours PO/IV
Prokinetic agents	Metoclopramide hydrochloride	0.1 to 0.3 mg/kg/dose to max 0.5 mg/kg/dose q 6 to 8 hours PO,IV ac
	Bethanechol chloride	0.1 to 0.2 mg/kg/dose PO q 6 to 8 hours ac
	Cisapride	0.1 to 0.3 mg/kg/dose PO q 6 to 8 hours
Anticholestasis agents	Ursodiol (UDCA)	7.5 to 22.5 mg/kg/dose q 12 hours (stable in solution for 5 days after preparation)

Gastrointestinal Support of Feeding Problems
Feeding Intolerance

The most common problem encountered when feeding very LBW infants is feeding intolerance. Markers commonly used to evaluate this problem include the quantity of gastric residuals, incidence of emesis, and pattern of stooling. Signs of intolerance are residuals that are green, bloody, or greater than one half of the previous 3 hours' intake. *Any* occurrence of emesis is a concern, and the infant should be assessed.

A minimum initial evaluation should include an examination of the abdomen, the feeding tube placement, the baby's position, and a review of the child's medications. Stools that become frequent, loose, contain glucose, or have a low pH (<5.5) signal a need for evaluation for sepsis or intolerance of milk or medications.

If the initial evaluation is unremarkable, consideration should be given to decreasing the volume of feeds, changing the strength or type of milk, or changing the mode of feeding to a milk drip or a slow infusion over 60 to 120 minutes. Babies who have glucose-positive or acidic stools who are shown to be sepsis free should be investigated for the presence of malabsorption.

Gastroesophageal Reflux

Because of esophageal, antral, or duodenal dysfunction, many infants with chronic lung disease develop gastroesophageal reflux (GER). Although lower esophageal sphincter tone is decreased in preterm infants compared with term infants, GER in preterm infants appears to be related to delayed gastric emptying or abnormal duodenal activity. In addition, many congenital and acquired structural abnormalities of the gastrointestinal (GI) tract can present with vomiting. Thus, the initial evaluation of the infant with GER should include a barium swallow with visualization of the upper GI tract. Because this radiographic study is performed under stressful artificial circumstances, it is not an adequate method to evaluate lower esophageal sphincter tone. If there are no anomalies and clinical evidence of reflux is present, a trial of H_2 antagonists or prokinetic agents is warranted (Table 10).

Intestinal Dysmotility

Delayed intestinal transit of nutrients is demonstrated by the presence of increased abdominal girth and poor stool output with or without the presence of gastric residuals. Better intestinal motor activity may be achieved by feeding full-strength, rather than dilute, formulas. Cereal or fiber may also enhance antral and intestinal motor activity, and prokinetic agents may improve transit (Table 10).

Ineffective Sucking

Although the sucking mechanism is present at 32 to 34 weeks' gestation, many infants who have chronic lung disease have difficulty sucking. Effective propulsion of oral nutrients requires that an infant exert both a coordinated effort and adequate strength of effort. To allow the baby adequate sucking opportunity for development of the skill of sucking, infants should be periodically offered 'pacifier practice,' or experience with nonnutritive sucking, beginning at 32 to 34 weeks' gestation. Infants who have difficulty establishing sucking skills may benefit from occupational therapy and speech pathology consultation and the establishment of a consistent feeding regimen.

Short Gut

Chronic inflammation, bacterial overgrowth, and malabsorption may occur in bowel-recovering NEC or surgical resection. The presence of acidic, glucose-positive stools and increased frequency or volume of stools may indicate that any or all of these problems exist. Smaller volume of milk drip feedings is frequently helpful. The clinician should consider zinc supplements and carefully follow protein nutrition laboratory values while maximizing protein delivery. Generally, it is more desirable in premature infants to continue using premature formulas; however, in some cases, predigested formulas are needed but may be a nutritional compromise. If intolerance persists when predigested formulas are fed, subspecialty consultation may be helpful.

Cholestasis

Cholestasis may occur in infants who have received chronic TPN. Introduction of small enteral feedings and decreased use of TPN may be helpful in reversing or reducing progression of cholestasis. Pharmacologic agents (Table 10) may also enhance hepatic clearance of bilirubin and reduce cholestasis.

By Virginia F. Schneider, PA-C, and Carol L. Berseth, MD

Suggested Reading

Anderson DM, Kliegman RM: The relationship of neonatal alimentation practices to the occurrence of endemic necrotizing enterocolitis. *Am J Perinatol* 1991;8:62-67.

Anderson GC: Current knowledge about skin-to-skin (Kangaroo) care for preterm infants. *J Perinatol* 1991;11:216-226.

Biondillo (Hurst) N: *Breast-Feeding Your Hospitalized Baby.* Houston, Texas Children's Hospital, 1988.

Blondheim O, Abbasi S, Fox WW, et al: Effect of enteral gavage feeding rate on pulmonary functions of very low birth weight infants. *J Pediatr* 1993;122:751-754.

Brown RL, Wessel J, Warner BW: Nutrition considerations in the neonatal extracorporeal life support patient. *Nutr Clin Pract* 1994;9:22-27.

Edelman NH, Rucker RB, Peavy HH: Nutrition and the respiratory system. *Am Rev Respir Dis 1986*;134:347-352.

Friedman Z, Rosenberg A: Abnormal lung surfactant related to essential fatty acid deficiency in a neonate. *Pediatrics* 1979;63:855-859.

Gibson AT, Pearse RG, Wales JKH: Knemometry and the assessment of growth in premature babies. *Arch Dis Child* 1993;69:498-504.

Grant J, Denne SC: Effect of intermittent versus continuous enteral feeding on energy expenditure in premature infants. *J Pediatr* 1991;118:928-932.

Hamill PV, Drizd TA, Johnson CL: Physical growth: National Center for Health Statistics percentiles. *Am J Clin Nutr* 1979;32:607-629.

Haumont D, Deckelbaum RJ, Richelle M, et al: Plasma lipid and plasma lipoprotein concentrations in low birth weight infants given parenteral nutrition with twenty or ten percent lipid emulsion. *J Pediatr* 1989;115:787.

Heird WC, Kashyap S, Gomez MR: Parenteral alimentation of the neonate. *Semin Perinatol* 1991;15:493-502.

Heldt GP: The effect of gavage feeding on the mechanics of the lung, chest wall, and diaphragm of preterm infants. *Pediatr Res* 1988;24:55-58.

Kurzner SI, Garg M, Bautista DB: Growth failure in infants with bronchopulmonary dysplasia: nutrition and elevated resting metabolic expenditure. *Pediatr* 1988;81:379-384.

Macdonald PD, Skeoch CH, Carse H, et al: Randomized trial of continuous nasogastric, bolus nasogastric, and transpyloric feeding in infants of birth weight under 1400 g. *Arch Dis Child* 1992;67:429-431.

Meetze WH, Valentine C, McGuigan JE, et al: Gastrointestinal priming prior to full enteral nutrition in very low birth weight infants. *J Pediatr Gastroenterol Nutr* 1992;15:163-170.

Morales E, Craig LD, MacLean WC Jr: Dietary management of malnourished children with a new enteral feeding. *J Am Diet Assoc* 1991;91:1233.

Moskowitz SR, Pereira G, Spitzer A, et al: Prealbumin as a biochemical marker of nutritional adequacy in premature infants. *J Pediatr* 1983; 102:749-753.

Neu J, Valentine C, Meetze W: Scientifically-based strategies for nutrition of the high-risk low birth weight infant. *Eur J Pediatr* 1990;150:2-13.

Orenstein SR: Controversies in pediatric gastroesophageal reflux. *J Pediatr Gastroenterol Nutr* 1992;14:338.

Rivera A Jr, Bell EF, Bier DM: Effect of intravenous amino acids on protein metabolism of preterm infants during the first three days of life. *Pediatr Res* 1993;33:106–111.

Schanler RJ: Suitability of human milk for the low-birthweight infant. *Clin Perinatol* 1995;22:207-222.

Sondheimer JM: Gastroesophageal reflux: update on pathogenesis and diagnosis. *Pediatr Clin North Am* 1988;35:103.

Sosenko IRS, Frank L: Nutritional influences on lung development and protection against chronic lung disease. *Semin Perinatol* 1991;15:462-468.

Valentine CJ, Hurst NM, Schanler RJ: Hindmilk improves weight gain in low birth weight infants fed human milk. *J Pediatr Gastroenterol Nutr* 1994;18:474-477.

Vanderhoff JA: Short bowel syndrome. *Clin Perinatol* 1996;23:377-386.

Yunis KA, Oh W: Effects of intravenous glucose loading on oxygen consumption, carbon dioxide production, and resting energy expenditure in infants with bronchopulmonary dysplasia. *J Pediatr* 1989;115: 127-132.

Chapter 12

Ethical Considerations

Parent-Physician Communication

Effective communication serves as a major cornerstone of support for parents during an infant's hospitalization. Initial parent-physician encounters are often limited to quick, informal discussions. But as soon as the infant is relatively stable, the physician should meet formally with the parents to achieve these goals: (1) to educate the parents in a general manner about their child's illness; (2) to identify the personal needs of the family and of others who may provide emotional support; (3) to clarify expectations for future communication and decision-making, and to identify key neonatal intensive care unit (NICU) personnel to the family; and (4) to demonstrate empathy and compassion. These formal meetings should occur in a calm environment away from the bedside to permit the parents and the physician to focus on the discussion; this is especially important for the initial encounter, because this sets an important tone for the parent-physician interaction for the duration of the infant's hospitalization.

The acuity of the infant's care often determines the style of ongoing communication adopted by parents and the physician. Although communication can be provided informally by others caring for the infant, the physician should maintain consistent rapport with the family to ensure that accurate information is conveyed and to establish a sense of constancy and trust. Furthermore, the neonatologist must communicate with the infant's obstetrician and primary care pediatrician, because they often provide the family support while the infant is acutely ill.

Table 1: Suggested Readings for Parents of Premature Infants

- Harrison H, Kositsky A: *The Premature Baby Book: A Parents Guide to Coping and Caring in the First Years*. New York, St Martin's Press, 1983.

- Manginello FP, DiGeronimo TF: *Your Premature Baby. Everything You Need to Know About the Childbirth, Treatment, and Parenting of Premature Infants*. New York, John Wiley & Sons Inc, 1991.

- Shelov SP, Hannemann RE: *Caring for Your Baby and Young Child*. New York, Bantam Books, 1983.

- Dewyze J: *The Baby Came Early: A Moving Account of the Premature Birth of Her Child*. Ben-Simon Publications, 1986.

- Lafferty LES: *Born Early: A Premature Baby's Story for Children*. Songbird Publications, 1994.

- Murphy-Melas E, Tate D: *Watching Bradley Grow: A Story About Premature Birth*. Longstreet Press, 1996.

- Gotsch G: *Breastfeeding Your Premature Baby*. La Leche League International, 1990.

The physician should recognize that the family can develop any number of coping styles. Some may remain aloof, others may become confrontational, and still others may become overly dependent on caregivers. Although these adaptive styles may make communication difficult for the physician, consistent, ongoing interaction with the family should remain a priority in the daily care of the infant.

Extended family and friends can provide important support to the family. Family support should be buttressed by pastoral support, peer-support groups, social workers, and the infant's primary care providers. Personal family physicians can often provide additional background information and 'translate' technical concepts. A library of consumer-oriented information is often available (Table 1).

Prenatal Counseling and Delivery Room Care

Many high-risk deliveries are identified prenatally, and neonatologists may be asked to provide consultation or parental education, or to assist in decision-making. When delivery is imminent, the physician's role is to prepare the family for the events that are anticipated at birth. Families may also wish to provide the neonatologist with specific directives about the extent of delivery room care for their infant. *However, the physician should not make a commitment to the family to resuscitate or to withhold resuscitation until the infant can be evaluated.*

Withholding Care
Do-Not-Resuscitate Orders

The process of informed consent requires that decision-making be done in consultation with the family. These conversations should be routinely documented in the medical record. When the physician and parents agree that resuscitation should not be provided to an infant if cardiac arrest occurs, a note must be written in the chart attesting to the virtual futility of the infant's survival. Orders not to resuscitate the infant must be written in the chart by the attending physician and communicated to the staff. It should be emphasized to families that a do-not-resuscitate (DNR) order pertains only to this single aspect of care, and that attention to other needs will continue to be provided.

Occasionally, parents and physicians disagree about treatment plans. It is important that physicians thoroughly discuss their decision-making process with families and offer consultation for second opinions. Most pediatric hospitals offer consultation services to assist families and physicians in resolving these conflicts. Others maintain guidelines and procedures to identify when ongoing care is futile or inappropriate. While committee decisions and futility guidelines are not legally binding, formal case review can give family members an opportunity to vent their frustrations and permit the establishment of consensus.

Withdrawing Life Support

Ideally, an atmosphere should be created that recognizes the dignity of the patient, minimizes the suffering of the infant, and provides emotional support for the family. The dying infant should be relieved of pain, and unnecessary support should be discontinued. Parents should be able to choose whether they prefer to be with the child in a private, hospice-like environment or to remain within the mainstream of the NICU. In addition, parents should participate in decisions concerning withdrawal of support (eg, ventilator). Regardless of the manner chosen for the infant to die, the process should be unhurried and orderly.

When an infant dies, several administrative details must be completed. Generally, families must be asked to consider organ donation and autopsy and to designate funeral arrangements. The physician must write a death note in the chart, designate the time of death, and complete the death certificate.

Questions and issues concerning the infant's care may continue after death. Therefore, posthumous contact is essential and can be provided by nurses, neonatologists, or family physicians by telephone or formal interview. If the grieving process appears to be dysfunctional, referral for counseling may be offered.

By Carol L. Berseth, MD, and Timothy R. Cooper, MD

Suggested Reading

American Academy of Pediatrics Committee on Bioethics. Ethics and the care of critically ill infants and children. *Pediatrics* 1996;98:149-152.

Berseth CL: Ethical dilemmas in the neonatal intensive care unit. *Mayo Clin Proc* 1987;62:67-72.

Brent DA: A death in the family: the pediatrician's role. *Pediatrics* 1983;72:645-651.

Evans AL, Brody BA: The do-not-resuscitate order in teaching hospitals. *JAMA* 1985;253:2236-2239.

Fost N, Crawford RE: Hospital ethics committees. Administrative aspects. *JAMA* 1985;253:2687-2692.

Halevy A, Brody BA: Brain death: reconciling definitions, criteria, and tests. *Ann Intern Med* 1993;119:519-525.

Halevy A, Brody BA: A multi-institution collaborative policy on medical futility. *JAMA* 1996;276:571-574.

Schneidarman LJ, Jecker NS, Johnsen AR: Medical futility: its meaning and ethical implications. *Ann Intern Med* 1990;112:949-954.

Chapter 13

Discharge Planning

Discharge Criteria

Every discharge must be considered individually and active problems should be resolved or managed through outpatient care. Nevertheless, guidelines for discharge may be helpful. The following are minimum criteria for discharge:

1. Parents or guardians are willing and capable of taking care of the baby and the home environment is stable.
2. Parents and caretakers demonstrate competence performing normal care of the infant. They must be trained to anticipate signs and symptoms of illness and respiratory decompensation, and they should demonstrate adequate skills in operating equipment and performing anticipated emergency procedures (eg, cardiopulmonary resuscitation [CPR]).
3. The baby must be stable for at least 1 to 2 weeks, without significant changes in medication or ventilatory support. If on oxygen, the baby must be able to recover quickly from brief periods in room air, which will invariably occur at home.
4. The baby must have evidence of adequate nutritional intake and growth.

Table 1 is meant to be a guide for discharging an infant with chronic lung disease but is by no means exhaustive.

Home Apnea Monitoring

Home monitoring is one of the most controversial issues in neonatology. There is no consistent, universally accepted standard of care outlining which infants should receive home apnea

Table 1:	Discharge Checklist for Chronic Pulmonary Disease
Medical support	Identify the primary care physician
	Follow up with pulmonary specialist 1 to 2 weeks after discharge
	Follow up with developmental specialist 1 to 2 months after discharge
	Bring immunizations current, including influenza and pneumococcus
Home nursing therapy	Arrange frequently in the beginning (several times a week to 24-hour care); wean as family gains skills and confidence
Home respiratory therapy	Arrange nebulizer treatments and equipment
	Arrange home ventilator and monitoring equipment

monitoring. About 8% to 10% of infants discharged from the neonatal intensive care unit are sent home on apnea monitors.

The National Institutes of Health Consensus Conference on Infantile Apnea and Home Monitoring does not recommend routine monitoring or screening of normal term or preterm infants.

Home monitoring is usually considered in these situations (Table 2): persistent apnea, an apparent life-threatening event (ALTE), and selected infants with a history of apnea of pre-

Table 2: Recommendations for Home Apnea Monitoring and CPR Training

- Persistent, symptomatic apnea in premature infants
- History of a severe ALTE or apneic episode
- Sibling or twin of a SIDS* victim
- The technology-dependent child, such as infants requiring mechanical ventilation
- Severe feeding difficulties with gastroesophageal reflux with apnea and bradycardia
- The child with pulmonary, cardiac, or neurologic problems such as bronchopulmonary dysplasia requiring oxygen supplementation, tracheostomies, or central hypoventilation
- Abnormal multichannel recording documenting significant apnea and increased periodic breathing

* Sudden infant death syndrome

maturity. The relationship between apnea of prematurity and infantile apnea is unclear. The benefit from home apnea monitoring appears to be the poorest in infants whose apnea of prematurity appears to have resolved. While apnea of prematurity usually resolves by 36 weeks' postmenstrual age (see *Control of Breathing*, Chapter 9), some premature infants continue to have idiopathic apnea at this age, when they are otherwise ready for discharge. Infants discharged on home oxygen may benefit as well. The monitor may provide warning should the nasal cannula become dislodged and the infant subsequently develops apnea. Infants with ALTE may also benefit from being monitored.

The effectiveness of home apnea monitoring in reducing infant mortality and morbidity is not established, although experience suggests that apnea monitoring may be effective in certain infants that are at an extraordinary risk of dying. Nonetheless, monitoring cannot guarantee survival. Compliance with monitor use has been shown to be poor. Recording monitors document and encourage use as well as aid in interpretation of alarm situations.

Observation of premature infants in a standard car safety seat before hospital discharge is recommended to monitor for possible apnea, bradycardia, or oxygen desaturation. If any of these events occur, equipment placing the infant in a semiupright position should be avoided, and alternative child restraint devices should be discussed with the family before discharge.

Home oxygen: See BPD, Chapter 5.

Respiratory Syncytial Virus Prophylaxis

Now approved by the FDA, respiratory syncytial virus immune globulin intravenous (RespiGam™) has been shown to reduce morbidity and hospitalization of high-risk infants acquiring RSV infection. The American Academy of Pediatrics recommendations for use of RSV-IGIV are complex and should be reviewed for specific guidelines for individual patients before initiating therapy. The recommendations are:

- Prophylaxis should be considered for infants and children less than 2 years of age with bronchopulmonary dysplasia who are receiving or have received oxygen therapy in the past 6 months before the start of the regional RSV season.
- Infants born at less than 32 weeks' gestation.
- Prophylaxis should be initiated before the regional onset of RSV season and continued monthly to the end of the regional season at 750 mg/kg/dose.
- Educating parents and caregivers about infection control and respiratory disease risk prevention is a key adjuvant to RSV-IGIV prophylaxis.
- Because prophylaxis is costly and administration logistically demanding, the cost effectiveness and feasibility

of use in individual patients should be evaluated by child health-care providers.

Immunization with measles-containing vaccines may be delayed for 9 months after the last dose of RSV-IGV. Other standard immunizations should be given routinely. Use has not been approved for infants with congenital heart disease (CHD), although there may be indications for use in preterm infants with asymptomatic cyanotic CHD.

Home Nutrition

Home nutrition is an extension of the plan begun in the hospital. When discharging on special diets, effective education of the parents about the reasons for dietary restriction is the best method of ensuring compliance. The clinician should schedule frequent weight checks to demonstrate continued growth and to reassure parents. The availability of special formulas in the community should be assessed. Invariably, supplies run out unexpectedly, and substitution may be required. If the child is on a formula that may not be readily available on short notice, the clinician should suggest alternatives. Vitamins and fluoride should be ordered if area water is inadequately supplemented. The clinician should order iron for anemic infants.

By Virginia F. Schneider, PA-C, Michelle M. Heng, MD, and Charleta Guillory, MD

Suggested Reading

American Academy of Pediatrics Committee on Infectious Diseases, Committe on Fetus and Newborn. Respiratory synctial virus immune globulin intravenous: indications for use. *Pediatrics* 1997;99:645-649.

American Academy of Pediatrics Committee on Injury and Poison Prevention and Committee on Fetus and Newborn. Safe transportation of premature and low birth weight infants. *Pediatrics* 1996;97:758-760.

Ballard RA: *Pediatric Care of the ICN Graduate.* Philadelphia, WB Saunders Co, 1988.

National Institutes of Health Consensus Development Conference on Infantile Apnea and Home Monitoring, Sept 29 to Oct 1, 1986. *Pediatrics* 1987;79:292-299.

Index

D

2,3-diphosphoglycerate (2,3-DPG) 22, 23

dead space ventilation 19

dead space volume 7, 19

dentition 239

dexamethasone 90, 160

dextrose 297

diabetes 46, 50, 51, 80, 96

diaphragm 3, 12, 55, 56, 217, 219

diaphragmatic agenesis 183

diaphragmatic hernia 53, 55, 100, 103, 114, 139, 171, 176, 178, 183, 225, 236, 242, 265, 269

diaphragmatic paralysis 191

diffusion block 27, 28

digitalis 116

dipalmitoyl phosphatidyl-choline (DPPC) 43-45

diphtheria 204

discharge criteria 311

discharge planning 154

distending pressure 8, 9, 64, 66-68

distention 201, 208

diuresis 85, 86

diuretics 99, 116

do-not-resuscitate (DNR) 308

docosahexaenoic acid (DHA) 294

dopamine 93, 106, 127, 191, 228

doxapram 215, 221

driving pressure [P(t)] 13

drug abuse 51

ductus arteriosus 33

dwarfism 182

dynamic lung compliance 68, 70

dysphagia 209

dyspnea 176

dystrophy 183

E

E coli 131, 132

echocardiogram 76

echocardiography 163

ectopia cordis 194

edema 86, 142, 216

electrocardiogram 179

electrolytes 283, 285

Ellis-van Creveld syndrome (chondroectodermal dysplasia) 182, 195

emesis 302

emphysema 3, 4, 39, 55, 140-142, 165, 172, 173, 176, 204

encephalopathy 202, 203

end expiration 15

end inspiration 15, 19

endotracheal tube 63, 65

Enfamil® 292, 293

W

X

Z